SEWING SEQUINS ON MY STRAIGHT JACKET

A HEARTWARMING AND HONEST MEMOIR .

SHARON COOK

Published by SpellBound Books 2024

To H, Pops, Tam, Sam and Olly

x

To Della –
really hope you laugh
x ... Thank you –
you have been a part
of this journey!
love
[illegible]
xxx

FOREWORD

Sometimes I miss them, when they're asleep, even after the worst of days. The days you think will never end, the days you can't think, can't pee, can't even drink tepid coffee. Yet I wished they could be little for ever. At least I could protect them from the harsh world, a world where people will take from them, hurt them, ridicule them and steal their innocence.

Then again, as their mum and protector, I have to prepare them for the reality of a society that can't wait to guzzle them up and spit them out, like a piece of chewing gum which has lost its zing.

We have had a rough ride these last few years. It has been a struggle to function on the most basic of levels. Looking back, I realise how tough it has been. We three have each lost out. Not because we have lost a husband and a father, to divorce. He was there at both conceptions, but he was never with us as part of the family. He was simply unable to give anything back.

I think I miss them when they are asleep because their absence means I can be who I once was. There is calm, there is peace, there is time to think. I can focus on what my life has become, how it is so different to what it was before, how it is nothing like I imagined yet it contains one of the things I wanted more than anything else in the world – children.

Here I am. A 'geriatric' mum. I have two children. It's miraculous they were born at all. I love them. I know it's not all *Little House on the Prairie,* believe me, I know it's not all cotton candy and starched white aprons.

Sometimes I have to go and check on them when they are asleep, check they are still breathing, look at them, remind myself being on my own with them is OK. Then, when I go downstairs, I miss them and it is almost painful. I tell myself I am not lonely. I know being a single mum is not the end of the world.

When I am calm and not distracted by a bone weariness so acute I can barely walk, I want to be with them, grow and learn with them, laugh with them. I want us to enjoy the life we have, the life we will build. When we reach that point, the pain will lessen.

And when I wrote all that, it never occurred to me either of my children would get cancer.

CHAPTER ONE

It was the first time in my life I had not been able to open my own front door.

On that wet and wild night I was shaking so much I couldn't wiggle the key properly. My neighbour had to do it for me.

With a hand on my shoulder, she gently pushed me over the tiny threshold.

'Just pack what you can carry,' she said. 'Do you have a couple of bags to hand? I can get you some.'

Shaking my head, I told her I'd be fine. Fine? What did that mean – fine? What was I saying? She agreed to come back in half an hour.

'Becky, can you follow me and if I give you my car keys can you get it back here for me? I'm really sorry to ask but I don't know what to do with the car.'

'Don't be daft,' she said, 'I'll drive you. Now go and pack. Just take what you need. Plenty of pyjamas! And don't forget clean knickers – and toothbrushes for all of you.'

I went upstairs, remembering earlier in the day how my son had got stuck half way up – or was it half way down? The Grand Old Duke of York hadn't been much help.

'I can't move mummy, I'm stuck. It hurts mummy, it hurts. It really hurts. I can't move.'

Moments earlier I had been shouting at him to get ready; we had to go feed the chickens. 'Get your wellies on!' I'd hollered.

'Mummy I can't move, it hurts. It really, really hurts.'

Did I feel the fear then? Did my son's bleats of pain from this morning warn me of the horror to come? And tell me, how can a few hours change a life so utterly and completely you feel like you're walking in someone else's shoes?

I have minutes to pack all the things we would need for the next two weeks. Would it be two weeks? It could be two months. Longer? No one could tell me.

Is this what a refugee feels like when someone charges through the village shouting *'the soldiers are coming. Run!'*.

I wanted to run. I wanted to carry on running towards the horizon and not stop and not look back and just keep running as I fought to hang on to our old life. I wanted to run to keep up with my previous life, to grab it by the shirt tails and not let it go. I wanted the life I had yesterday, not the one promised for tomorrow by today's terrifying events.

But I couldn't run up the road screaming.

Minutes to pack two bags with some clothes and essentials to get my family through days? Weeks? Months?

At the top of the stairs, I noticed how tatty the carpet looked. Our black cat, Oscar Wilde, used the corner as a scratch pad, kitten Ruby Tuesday's black hairs seemed to pepper the landing from every angle.

The children's bedroom was willing me to make haste, the sight of their things – for once tidy rows of books, a pile of clean clothes on the corner of my son's bed, toys they had been playing with that morning – made me want to cry.

But there wasn't time, I had to move fast! But no running.

I grabbed a black leather travel bag from under my bed,

bought within sight of the Leaning Tower of Pisa, and started stuffing it with underwear, clothes, favourite books, socks – of course trying to find the pairs without holes!

Pens and pencils, the Nintendo DS, a bendy green dinosaur who *loved* cooking, a couple of our Tibetan blankets, toiletries – shoes, don't forget shoes and slipper socks and some hats and scarves and where are the gloves?

Into the bathroom, where's the purple plastic soap dish? Take a fresh soap, grab the new toothpaste, *Rescue Remedy* – must find the *Rescue Remedy*. I really must find the *Rescue Remedy*. Could it possibly help? Was it worth scrabbling around for some flower essences steeped in brandy? Maybe a large brandy would be more helpful? But there was no time, nor the inclination, to grab a stiff one.

Hair clips, couldn't go without those my hair desperately needed a cut, what clothes should I take? Had to find things that weren't full of holes – that'll do if I grab my sewing kit, I can repair it while I'm sat there. Can I wear that top with those jeans or will my belly show up too much?

Well, what is *de rigueur* for a hospital bedside?

My son lay in a hospital bed and I was fussing about what colour lacy vests to pack. What kind of mother was I? The kind who was losing the plot, that's the kind. Think fast, pack quicker, get back to my children. Running not allowed.

I took a last look around my cluttered bedroom – books everywhere, half-worn clothes draped on a paint-splattered chair, fabric, quilting magazines mingling with paperwork, earrings on top of stuff, stuff on top of stuff. When would I see my bed again, it's beautiful, curled bedstead such a feature? I had worked so hard for that bedstead. It was made to order and at the last minute I had wondered if it was too big for such a small cottage yet it had fitted, perfectly.

On the bed, unmade, a hideous furry blanket gifted by a

grandma used only because my son had been sick on the duvet the day before. Should I draw the curtains? How long would we be gone? I left my room looking like a troupe of Devonshire pixies had partied in it.

I grabbed Hornsly, a blue and maroon furry dinosaur, from H's bed. My son, who had turned nine just three days ago, wasn't in to dinosaurs particularly yet the two toys I packed for him were both prehistoric creatures. Dead for eons yet dinosaurs are a part of our reality today. Dead creatures. Oh God. Death.

Please don't let my son die. Who was I asking?

'How're you getting on?' Becky's voice cut through my brain wobble. 'Shall I put those in the car?' She pointed at the two bags in the hall before loading them in her car, just as I darted into the kitchen.

My kitchen was long and thin, hideous colours, part of the inherited fabric of our seventeenth century cottage. But I loved it, full of vintage china, a sturdy silver Kenwood mixer, grotty lino sporting damp stains harking back to the 1600's (or so it felt) – and a fridge loaded with the recent shop.

Oh no! What to do with a fridge full of food? Couldn't this have happened *before* I'd done a big shop, *before* I'd stocked the freezer? Why could this not have happened when I was about to hit the back of the cupboards, the moment you're down to a packet of dried asparagus soup past its sell by date and some weird flavoured oil bought at a food fair for three times its actual worth?

Food. What would we do for food in hospital? How would I feed us all? Would there be a kitchen, somewhere to cook?

'Becky, can you use this? Please, please use it. It'll go to waste otherwise.'

'You can use some of it,' she said.

I grabbed a carrier bag and filled it with apples, kiwi, a hunk of cheddar, bananas, cheesy biscuits, rice cakes, cereal bars and half a cucumber. Well, what do you take when you're fleeing your home?

The bag of Christmas shortbread, chocolate covered ginger biscuits and *Stollen* cakes sat quietly in the corner of the dining room, waiting to be remembered. The half dozen bottles of Glühwein looked on in icy silence. Still, at least they counted as some festive forward planning to come home to...

I glimpsed the pile of inedible gourds proudly displayed on our dining room table. I'd grown them from seed and just loved all the bobbly bits, some turning from green to a deep golden yellow, the white ones speckled with stripes of olive. All their little gnarled bits and twisted stems looked so perfect, autumnal and mystical. I was, for a moment, back in my old life, back in my childhood.

Reality hit as another thought crossed my jangled mind.

'Money,' I wailed. 'Becky, hang on. I need to sort out some money.'

Dashing upstairs, back the bedroom-come-home office I'd just said goodbye to – tripping over the fallen pile of books by my bed – I logged on and transferred two hundred pounds of meagre savings into a current account.

Dashing back downstairs, 'Can we stop at the cash point on the way out? I need some cash. And I'd better top up my mobile.'

Burbling like an idiot I got into Becky's people carrier, did up my seat belt.

'Becky, I need to get my address book. Sorry. Need to tell people and cancel a few things. Sorry.' I undid my seat belt and slipped out of the car door onto the sodden Tarmac. That hurt. All haste no speed, Grandma's words in my head. Be a bit rubbish if I beat my son to a hospital bed.

Grabbing last years' diary (I always seem to be a year behind...) and an address book we set off into the gales; weather and emotion in symbiosis, as turbulent outside as I felt inside.

How had I driven home earlier? It was a tree felling night, with added driving rain and pouring tears.

I don't remember much conversation on the way back to the hospital. Even for two of the chattiest of women there aren't many protocols for such situations.

All I could think was 'how do you tell your nine-year old son; 'You have cancer''?

CHAPTER
TWO

SAYING GOODBYE TO BECKY OUTSIDE THE MAIN ENTRANCE OF TORBAY Hospital, on the edge of the *English Riviera,* felt like saying goodbye to everything familiar, everything I knew, everything I had ever known.

I also felt fear. I knew this because I had felt it before, fleetingly, when I crossed the border into a war zone. That fear was brief. This one wasn't.

In the space of a few hours, in the time it took for a crisp autumn day to fade into a black, rain lashed night our 'new', old life was gone forever. I was carrying a bag in each hand, balancing one on my shoulder containing such essentials as half a cucumber, my handbag slung across the other shoulder. Only the thought of H and Pops in a hospital room propelled me forward.

Was I entering Narnia or crossing Hades? Nothing seemed real and the dark of the night, with no one around, added to the dream-like sense of everything unfolding. We hadn't just had the rug pulled from under us, someone had nicked the bloody house as well. No wardrobes to clamber through. You soon learn there are no wardrobes in hospital.

Back on the tatty-round-the-edges children's ward, I made

my way to the hospital room. H and Pops were in bed. I plonked down the bags, sat in the plastic covered institutional chair. Fortunately, we were in the right institution.

I must have sat, wrapped in silence, for some time. Reality seeped in. I needed the loo and set off to find the facilities. Seeing signs for the *Harrison Suite* pricked my memory.

Some months earlier Pops and I had been on the same ward. She had been admitted with acute appendicitis, plucked from what could have been a near-death experience by an eagle-eyed sonographer. Her words, 'book theatre NOW!' prompted a team of young surgeons to operate late on a Monday night. The same paediatric nurse who had checked Pops in, had also booked H in earlier. Had I been in poor taste, in the dying moments of our previous life back in A&E, when I joked my children were taking it in turns to get sick?

Pops' appendectomy was the reason I knew about the *Harrison Suite*. It was now far more poignant than last time – even though I knew it must be named after a dead person. I also knew it was a place I could get tea and coffee. I hoped it was empty.

On the way down the corridor a nurse hailed me. She had some blankets for us. As I thanked her, she put a hand on my arm.

'You know leukaemia treatments have really advanced in the last twenty years.' She smiled. I knew she was being kind. Did everyone on the ward know about H?

'And with this one he's got a sixty per cent chance of survival,' she babbled. 'So that's good, isn't it!?'

I couldn't talk, just mumbled something unintelligible and fled back to the room. Did I imagine that pitying look from the nurse on reception? Blanket nurse must have been absent for the lecture on 'being tactful with parents whose child has just been diagnosed with cancer'.

Survival rates. Survival rates! Oh my God. People were actually talking in terms of survival. A sixty per cent chance of survival meant he had a forty per cent chance of dying. Forty per cent!

What had the doctor said earlier? I had tried so hard to take everything in. I knew before I was taken to the little room, the little room with the standard issue box of tissues placed on a low table – the ones just a little bit too thin to be effective, but kinder on the budget. I knew the tall, kind-faced German consultant was going to tell me H had leukaemia because I had overheard some of the conversations back on A&E. And I had seen the panic on the face of the young, dark-haired house doctor as she tried to avoid my eyes, each time I asked her what was happening. I knew my son was very ill. Blanket nurse had voiced the statistics I had not been able to process. He could actually die.

Ever so gently the German consultant had told me, before I drove home to panic pack, they were not sure if H had Acute Lymphatic Leukaemia (ALL) or Acute Myeloid Leukaemia (AML), which was very aggressive and rare in children. Bound to be the rare one, I thought. He said we would have to go to Bristol Children's Hospital, where H would be assessed by specialists. Both involved chemotherapy, though AML would take around six months to treat, while ALL was treated over three years.

I had blurted out *'well, I hope it's AML, it'll be over more quickly'*. Looks were exchanged between the German consultant, the young dark-haired house doctor and a nameless nurse, who was probably in the room in case I needed attention. I didn't realise they meant H would be an in-patient for six months. I didn't know he could not be treated for AML in Devon. I didn't know a fungus could kill him. I did not know a lot of things back then.

Yes, I was told, H would lose his hair. He may need a heart transplant. The cancer was aggressive, so the treatment had to be too. How many *full siblings* did H have, in case he needed a bone marrow transplant? And yes, my son was very ill and was likely to get much sicker before we were able to go home.

'So, does that mean he doesn't have swine flu?' I asked. Everyone seemed to shift about uncomfortably.

'He will be assessed in Bristol,' said the kind German, clearly unprepared to discuss that scenario.

'I can drive us to Bristol in the morning,' I said. 'Will it be OK to wait until tomorrow, rather than set off now?'

This time I did not imagine the uncomfortable seat shifting. Gently and firmly the doctor explained it would be best for me not to drive to Bristol because there would be nowhere to park the car. They would arrange transport, in an ambulance.

'And Pops,' I said. Everyone shifted about. I was told they would *'make arrangements'.*

'Try and get some sleep' said nameless nurse. 'We'll start H on some treatment, start to prepare him.' I resisted the urge to let them know he wasn't an oven-ready chicken. My sense of humour was at death's door.

'First of all,' said the German consultant, 'we will need to secure him a bed in Bristol.'

'What if you can't?'.

'Then it might have to be Southampton. Or Oxford. Maybe Cardiff,' he said.

Walking back to the room then, before my dash home to panic pack, I had tried not to cry. I had actually pinched myself, hard on my left arm. There was no escape from this unfolding nightmare yet it didn't feel real. Hours later, sat in that horrible chair as my children slept, I felt the earlier pinch on my arm and noticed a bruise starting to show.

'Come on, girl,' said a quiet inner voice. *'Coffee! Find the Harrison Suite.'* For the second time that evening I wandered off in search of facilities. I also had to make phone calls. Other people needed to know H was ill. And I had to get practical. This was no time to start crying. It was time to make lists.

As I followed signs to the *Harrison Suite* I hoped no one else was around, but I was out of luck. A young couple were talking in hushed tones, obviously upset. I had no idea what they were going through, but I did hear them tell someone on the phone they'd be home the next day.

I felt devoid of compassion, couldn't smile at them and made a disgusting coffee using cheap instant granules all the while hoping they would leave. I saw the sign asking for a financial contribution to the tea and coffee, noted the mess in the sink. Dirty mugs, spilt milk, grotty screwed up paper towels, sugar melded to the caffeine-stained worktop. I washed up instead of giving money, in the selfish hope the young couple would go. They looked at me as if I was bonkers when I used the bleach I found under the sink. They left, leaving behind two unwashed mugs.

I dialled my parents, wondering how much credit I had left.

'Mum, hi, it's me. Look I don't have much time to talk but you both need to listen very carefully.' (Of course, I resisted the urge to say, 'I will zay zis only once'. My mum wouldn't have got the joke anyway).

It was just as hideous a phone call as you can imagine. I kept calm, told them very matter-of-factly their first grandchild, their only grandson, had cancer. I managed to say he would have to be in hospital for some time, probably in Bristol.

'Yes mum, he will have to have chemotherapy. Yes, I know it will be hard for him to lose his hair but they're telling me it is treatable.'

I found myself using the word *'treatable'* over and over. I was telling myself as much as them. 'Treatable, yes, treatable. He is very ill Mum. Yes, he will get very sick but there are drugs for that too.'

My mother was tearful, my father pragmatic.

'Tell us what we can do. Keep us informed,' he said. It was one of the last meaningful conversations I ever had with my dad.

It was getting late. I couldn't make any more phone calls. Just as I thought I was going to burst into tears, someone else came in to make a hot drink, and made some comment about me washing up. I must have grunted back before leaving the room, which was definitely suffering from delusions of grandeur. '*Suite*' my arse! It was small, full of insipid public information posters which begged to be ignored and stained hand written notes, taped to every available space, asking people to clear up after themselves.

It underlined how much I hated being trapped in faceless institutions, bombarded by ineffective signs telling me to conform, the straight lines of it all devoid of imagination. Still, it's not often you feel rebellious washing up a few mugs.

Wandering back to the room, seeing my children asleep, I knew I had to work out how to tell them H had cancer. I had to tell them the following morning. I would have to be honest, without scaring them.

I arranged some of the blankets, given by blanket nurse, on the floor and laid down by H's bed, stretched my legs out underneath Pops' pull-down bed. My head was pounding, my body ached and my tongue felt thick. Was I hot or cold, sweating or shivering? Must be shock, I thought. Day mingled with the longest of nights and as dawn streaked through the sky, the jolly, hideous curtains – at least half a meter too short for the windows – failed to shut out either Monday morning or the concrete of another hospital block.

Today I would have to deliver really bad news to an awful lot of people, with a stinking headache. At least no one would be able to smell my dog breath down the phone.

CHAPTER THREE

H HAD BEEN CLOSELY MONITORED THROUGHOUT THE NIGHT AND WAS hooked up to a syringe driver containing Calpol. His temperature had soared, not helped by me who had covered him in one of our Tibetan blankets when he started shivering.

'You do know,' said new morning shift nurse, 'that shivering is the body's way of trying to cool down, don't you?'

'So I've actually made him worse?' I said, horrified. Looked like it would be a while before I became Nurse Mum of the Year... New morning shift nurse shook her head and asked if either of the children wanted any toast. Pops nodded. H lay there looking pale and wan. Hell, he was pale and wan.

I perched on the side of H's bed.

'I need to talk to you both, about what's happening,' I managed to say, before feeling my throat tighten and a hot fuzz assaulting the back of my eyes.

'But first, you need toast and I need coffee. H, you sure you don't want any toast?'

I scuttled out of the room and into a loo, splashed my face with cold water and headed off in search of coffee.

Somehow, I managed to make it sound like we were off on

another adventure. When I said we would have to go in an ambulance – the first time for any of us – Pops asked if we could have blue flashing lights. *'Please don't let it be that bad,'* I thought, hoping my face didn't show the fear I felt.

'Look you two,' I said, knowing I couldn't cry. This had to sound as if I knew exactly what was happening. I had to control my own feelings in order to reassure the children everything was fine. 'We all need to know H is a very poorly boy. We're going to a special hospital for children, in Bristol.' *Well, hopefully Bristol...*

'Where's Bristol?' asked Pops.

'Err... It's up the motorway. It's where we get off the M5 and onto the M4, when we go back to Reading,' I said. Pops was pretty good with her roads.

'So, you mean its half way between where we live now and where we used to live, where we were born?' said Pops.

'Yup, you've got it,' I said, realising she was absolutely right. We would be exactly half way between the two towns we knew best in the world, though I hadn't ever 'been' to Bristol, only ever passed through it.

I kept telling the children not to worry; it would mean time off school for both of them. I chose my words carefully and reasoned I had to be straight; it would be far worse for either of them to overhear anything and not understand what was happening. I did not want them to get frightened. I had always tried to be honest with my children, answer questions directly, while respecting their childhood. Here goes...

'H, you have something called leukaemia, it's turned your blood a bit crazy. And leukaemia is a type of cancer of the blood,' I said.

'I've got cancer?' said H. Pops' eyes bulged.

'But mum,' he said, 'that's not good, is it?'

'No love, it's not very good. You are a very sick boy. But the good bit is the doctors know what it is and they will be able to sort it all out,' I said, my tone of voice doing its best to sound convincing.

'Look love,' I said, directly to H, hoping my voice wasn't going to crack, begging the hot fuzz building behind my eyes not to break through. 'You are a very sick boy. We're going to be spending quite a bit of time in hospital and we'll get to meet loads of doctors and nurses. And you're going to have to take a lot of medicines and some of them will make you feel very ill. But we have to fight off this *Crazy Blood*. And we will!'

By then Pops was sat by me on H's bed, my arm around her.

'Mummy,' said H, 'I'm not going to die – am I?'

Now that particular page of *An Idiot's Guide to Parenting* had clearly been torn out of the manual, before I even got to not read it. I was faced with no choice whatsoever: I lied.

'No H, you will not die. You have cancer of the blood and you will have to take some pretty horrible drugs to make the *Crazy Blood* go away. But you will not die. And you've got me and Pops looking out for you as well. We'll both be with you every step of the way! 'Fraid you're stuck with us mister!'

H smiled. 'Thanks mum. I love you.' And he drifted off to sleep. Or was it unconsciousness?

I didn't have the heart to tell him on top of all that that he was going to lose all his dark, curly *surfer dude* hair. He was often mistaken for a girl, with such long hair, which always made him giggle. H was definitely in touch with his feminine side.

Well, what would you have done? I'd told far bigger whoppers - Father Christmas, the Easter Bunny and the Tooth Fairy – hadn't I? I had no choice. It was a lie – because I had no idea what the outcome would be. Would it be sixty per cent – or forty? No one knew if H was going to live or die. No one could know. The doctors couldn't tell me what kind of leukaemia H had. No one could even tell me where we would be sleeping that night. But you cannot tell your nine-year-old son he might die, you can't.

It was, however, becoming increasingly obvious H was not at all well. His temperature had rocketed again, because of the leukaemia. His symptoms had not been typical. He was not covered in bruises. There had been no clue what his bone marrow had been up to, spewing out the deformed white blood cells which were busy swamping his red blood cells, failing to carry vital oxygen around his weakened body.

A rare trip to our GP the week before had heralded a diagnosis of 'probable swine flu', and that had given me the heeby geebies. People were dying from swine flu, people who had underlying health conditions, young people with immature immune systems. Still, H probably didn't have swine flu. It will have been the leukaemia, not swine flu. Even we couldn't be that unlucky.

Nurses came and went, more Calpol was administered and a pre-chemo drug was pumped through him. It all started to become a bit of a blur of sympathetic looks, pitying asides and concerned words.

Pops was bemused – and full of questions. 'What is leukaemia? How do you catch it? Why has H got it?' she asked. 'How long will be away for? Oh mummy, who will feed the cats while we're away? And the chickens?' She was an inquisitive seven-year-old. All her questions were good ones. Most of them were shooting around my head too.

It was all so unreal. I was sat in a small hospital room with hideous curtains, a very sick son, a frightened daughter and half a cucumber. Not quite the start I'd envisaged for this week.

CHAPTER FOUR

One of the advantages of a 'possible swine flu' diagnosis meant we had our own hospital room. It was hardly peaceful, but I was able to start making mental lists and figure who must be called.

I needed to ring school, tell them H and Pops wouldn't be in that day. That day? Week? Month? How on earth could I describe the scenario when I really didn't have any answers myself? But school needed to know – and fast. Our home town is small, the school a microcosm. Becky would be asked straight away why we seemed to have disappeared and it wasn't fair to dump that on her.

I found a large, deserted playroom at the end of the corridor, worn toys piled up. I almost expected Woody from Toy Story to pop up with a wave and a hearty, 'It's Ok, leukaemia's treatable these days', before grinning, waving his cowboy hat and jumping out of the window. Oh yeah, the window that didn't open. Having given up on the disgusting coffee, I was now onto black tea, marginally better and fairly essential as my throat was rather dry and croaky, not quite countering the pounding head.

The school switchboard put me straight through to the head teacher, after I explained we were in Torbay Hospital and I needed to speak to him directly. The news I was about to deliver was pretty immense. I had no idea what to say. I just dived straight in.

'Oh, hi there. It's H and Pops' mum. Just a quick call to let you know H won't be at school for a few months....

'No easy way to say this. He's got cancer. Diagnosed yesterday. Pops won't be there for a while either. Don't know how long...

'Terrible shock, yes. Sorry to have to give you such news. Yes, we're in Torbay Hospital, yes, the Torquay one. Just waiting for the ambulance to another hospital – no, don't know where yet. Might be Bristol, could be ... No, not sure how long we'll be gone...

'It's leukaemia. No, don't know what type. Yes, he will lose all his hair. No, I don't think we will be back in time for Christmas.

'Yes, do send some homework...Thank you, yes, that's very kind. Yes, I'll keep you informed. As soon as I know, yes...'

It was all a blur. I had to choose my words carefully so as not to freak anyone out. I did it the way I knew best – humorously. Now that sounds wrong, doesn't it? I don't mean cancer is funny, let's all have a darn good laugh, what ho! Though it certainly has its moments. But by then I'd have tried anything to make the whole thing sound, well - not quite so bad.

'At least we've discovered the ultimate cure for nits' became my stock response, batting away the serious questions with a 'yes, as soon as I know I'll be in touch'. The hospital equivalent of '*whatever*'. Or any one of those meaningless phrases which have seeded themselves into conversation – '*at the end of the day*' or '*to be honest with you*'. With cancer, in hospital, you soon learn you can never really give answers to questions, whatever the time the day ceases to exist. The situation merely evolves. It's the way it is.

I had to ring their dad. There was no way of avoiding it being while he was at work. Taking a deep breath, I dialled his office number. I knew he hadn't really taken it in but I made sure he knew to call me any time with questions. I promised him as soon as I knew where we would be going, I'd call him back. He had never been very good with emotions. Or humour.

Next, I called my former brother-in-law and his wife. I knew 'other' grandma was on holiday in Spain. The last thing I wanted was to let her know before they returned. Her husband was ill. It would most likely be the last holiday they had together. I wanted her to be able to enjoy it, while they could. There was nothing she – or anyone else – could do about our situation and I knew I needed time to gather my thoughts, find out what was likely to happen. I also knew I couldn't face it if she decided to fly home early and pitched up at hospital. She was more unpredictable than a hurricane.

I explained my reasoning to them and they said they felt she should know. I asked them to please respect what I had asked, the situation was difficult enough as it was and I felt it would be best for me to explain everything to her when she was back in England, which was soon. At least, by then, I'd know where we would be and how long we may be in hospital. I added I had rung because I wanted them to be able to support her when she got back.

As I began working my way through a list scrawled from my address book, taking into account my diary so I could cancel things as well, my head began to buzz. It was becoming clear my 'little black book' – bought because it really was a 'little black book' and the whole idea had always tickled me – was going to take time to work through. Not because it was held together by an elastic band, which helped to anchor in all the scraps of paper and backs of torn envelopes, receipts, corners of flyers with scrawled numbers, emails, house numbers. But I began to realise just how many other lives we had become a part of. It was surreal. We had become the trapped fly in the centre of a spider's web. In order to survive I had to communicate with every line of the web to get help to loosen the constraints holding us in.

The nits line became embellished with: 'Yup, we've gone from swine flu to leukaemia. Not quite so fashionable now'. Maybe I was being inappropriate?

Until you have had to do it yourself it's hard to explain how difficult it is to tell other people someone you love has cancer. How can you tell people gently, minimise the shock? You hear yourself speaking, as if you are looking down from above. You get used to your own phraseology, after a few calls. It doesn't make it easier. You also hear the unasked questions. The biggest elephant in the room being, *'you mean he could die?'*.

Again, I kept hearing myself use the word *'Treatable. It's treatable'*.

After about half a dozen more phone calls I had to stop. I was becoming too tearful. It's hard taking on board other people's shock, finding ways of reassuring them everything will be OK, when you have no idea if it will or it won't. It's also hard doing this kind of thing on your own. And I needed to be with H and Pops. *Shoulders back and – 'smile!'* said a small voice from somewhere. I was greeted by yet another nurse checking H's temperature who must, quite frankly, have thought I was a grinning idiot. Let's hope she was only right on one count.

'Any news yet? Do we know if it's Bristol?'

She looked fairly blank. 'I'm sure as soon as they know, they'll tell you.'

Was I really that annoying? But I needed to know. I had a so much to 'sort'.

Another nurse appeared soon after, somehow more senior sounding.

'Just a couple of questions for you,' she smiled. It was a smile right out of the training manual, which said nothing more than *'let's be havin' your attention'*.

'I think the doctor did mention your son may need a bone marrow transplant,' she said. How many *full siblings* has H got?'

'It's just Pops,' I said.

'But do they share the same father?' she said.

'Err, yes!' I said. 'And do we know where we're going yet?' I must have glared at her. She seemed to hurry out of the room. I may be a single parent – through divorce, the thought etched in capitals – but that doesn't make me a tart as well. Calm down said rational brain. There is a very good reason for asking the question – it's not a personal judgement about my morals, or lack thereof.

My head was full of questions. With few answers. At no point did anyone ever suggest I *'phone a friend'*. No one seemed to wonder why I was there on my own, with two children. No one said anything about Pops being there. In fact, no one was saying much about anything at all. I could so use a hug.

Less than 24 hours ago I was a single mum-of-two, quietly getting on with my life, head down but not drowning. Well, mostly not.

Who could I get to look after the cats for a couple of weeks, months? Where on earth would we stay? I'd probably need to find a cheap B&B for a few nights, wherever we ended up, while we got sorted. Money would run out quite quickly. I'd need my car but how would I manage that? Would the cottage be OK while we were away? Had I left a window open? Could I ask Becky to water the plants?

My head ached. All my joints seemed to be on fire. Must be shock. Pops was very quiet and clingy, H drifting in and out. I felt overwhelmed. At least I was used to that feeling, used to 'coping' on my own. I'd become a single parent three weeks before Pops was born. I'd been on my own for seven-and-a-half years. My coping mechanisms were well developed, yet I couldn't deny I was feeling a tad out of my depth.

The phone rang. My parents. What's happening? 'I don't know yet. Yes, talk soon. And can you tell Neil for me. Thanks.'

Neil is my younger brother and only sibling. Siblings! I wish I'd had ten children. It would have upped H's chances.

I began to wonder how all three of us would get to wherever we were being sent. If it was going to be in the back of an ambulance, would they get both Pops and me in? Still, all the staff here knew it was three of us, so they must have figured that one into the equation. It surely won't have been the first time they'd faced a situation like this.

Pops was tucked up in the pull-down bed, clearly shattered. H was asleep. 'I'm just going to go and make a few more calls Lovey,' I said. 'Stay there, I won't be long.'

I needed to see if there was still a world outside and, passing the nurses station by the horizontal fish tank where the fish looked as confused as I felt, forced myself to ask, *'any news?'* Luckily the response was more sympathetic than stony - must have been a shift change.

I resisted the urge to shout at someone 'look, my son has just been diagnosed with an aggressive life-threatening cancer and I need to bloody well know what happens next!' I smiled, probably not in a sweet, alluring, cheer leader kind of way, and told the desk I was going outside for some air.

'I've got my mobile in case you have any news,' I added, unhopefully and unhelpfully. One of them did at least smile at me, in a 'we-do-understand-this-is-a difficult-situation-for-you' kind of way. It was a busy ward, as I had already experienced with Pops and her appendectomy, with plenty of families coming and going. Though I was getting the very distinct impression childhood cancer was not part of their remit. Was this why we were being shipped out so promptly? Cancer isn't contagious ...

I felt like I was walking away from one void, straight into another. Walking up long corridors, needlessly lit by huge overhead Neons, everyone was going about their business as if nothing had happened. Maybe they were patients, staff – most doctors don't seem to wear long white coats any more – consultants, cleaners. I could have walked past someone who had saved a life in an operating theatre, past someone whose partner had died, past a volunteer who had just sold a packet of crisps or past someone who had been diagnosed with cancer. I was as invisible as the rest of the world, my fear and confusion as hidden as that of the people I walked past. The world was still turning. Ours was turning upside down.

Approaching the main entrance, I found myself virtually running to the outside. I had to escape the claustrophobic, coffin-like confines of dirty white walls.

I knew if I walked past the main car park, half way down the hill on the left was a green area bordered by tall pine trees. I stepped off the pavement snaking its way to the bottom of the hill, past a wooden bench and stood, breathing in the metallic air, the coniferous tang tempered by car fumes.

Not caring if anyone else was about, I stood, staring up at the sky, feet slightly apart, arms out, hands pointing down. Was I attempting to centre myself with the earth's core, channel some Totnesian cancer-clearing vibe passed on by a yogic with seventeen generations worth of Native American healing lore? Well, Totnes wasn't that far from Torquay. If any town had an alternative answer it was the TQ-niners – as they are fondly known round here. Totnes, the spiritually funky health food capital of the developed world, with added chick peas and ginseng. Either way I felt I had to stand firm, in case I floated away. I felt all floaty, like a summer skirt, a piece of muslin drying on the line. Dreamlike. Life had become unreal, unattached, unknown. Even more untethered.

The day before, I had been screeching at my son to get his wellies on so we could go and feed the chickens. Less than a day had passed since he cried out in pain *'it hurts mummy, it hurts'*, the pain so bad he got stuck half way up the stairs. Twenty-four hours ago, we three had lives much like anyone else's. Eat, sleep, work, play, pay the bills. Since a Sunday telephone call to the out-of-hours doctor we had been passed from one hospital to another, who were now sending us to a third.

My son had cancer. My nine-year old son had cancer and now our lives had no shape at all, nothing to tether us to anything – or anybody.

I stood under a huge sky, tear ducts in overdrive. There are moments in life when time really does stand still. No slow motion, no flash backs. Just stillness. Literally the calm before the storm. Grasp those moments. It's often the only chance you ever get to tell yourself *'get on with it'*. There is no time for self-pity. I knew by then I wasn't just taking on H's cancer. I also had another battle: keeping the three of us together.

Taking a last few glugs of Devon air, I took a final look at the trees and the sky. I needed it just to get through the smokers on the way back into hospital. How I resisted the urge to tell them *'don't you know smoking gives you cancer?'* I really don't know.

Oh the irony and injustice of it all.

CHAPTER FIVE

It was Bristol! We were off to Bristol. Geographically it was the best place we could be. There was a bed available and the plan was to get us there that day.

By chance I was on one of my corridor walks, which beat just sitting in the room, waiting, when I saw two men in paramedic gear. One of the nurses on the station saw me, her look told me they were there for us. I think my sudden appearance had interrupted the conversation. Non-verbal communication can be so much louder than the spoken word.

Both men were tall. They had friendly faces and off-beat names. It became very evident no one had told them we were a trio. Communication, as I have learnt, is not a strong point within the NHS. Yet I did feel someone, somewhere, had figured these were exactly the men for the job.

It transpired H was so sick we had to travel with a Specialist Paediatric Resuscitation Nurse. It meant if his heart stopped beating or he became even sicker, en route, there was someone on hand to administer life-saving treatment – in addition to the paramedics. I refused to let the fear take over. Someone was still trying to source a fully stocked resuscitation pack. While that was being done – I'll call them Bill and Ben but don't be fooled, these two men were sharp – realised there was a second child in the equation.

I had anticipated the response and politely reminded the nursing staff that Pops was coming with us. I knew I had not imagined the paper shuffling on the nurse's station, the lack of eye contact, the subtle seat shifting. Bill and Ben looked at each other. Boy, were the non-verbals deafening.

'We can only take two, with the nurse in the back,' said the younger one.

'But there are three of us,' I said. 'I have two children.'

'Well...' said the older one, glancing at his colleague. 'There is a fold down seat. But the safety belt isn't working. If you're happy with that mum...?'

Mantra in head. *'I will not cry. I will not cry.'* I did my best to smile without crying, wiped away a tear and mumbled, *'thank you'.* I felt sure we would invalidate the insurance. I'm sure it broke all the rules. I am equally as sure they took in the situation for exactly what it was and, for a tiny moment, I didn't feel quite so alone.

The nursing staff had taken the ostrich approach, assumed I'd crash and burn at the last moment, give in over Pops. THEY REALY DIDN'T GET IT. Who can you call when there is no one you can call??? (Ghostbusters don't count). It underlined how insignificant we were; how alone I really was.

My synapses were aligning, battle lines appearing. That small yet huge act of kindness, by two paramedics I'd never met, was humbling. It gave me more insight into what I was facing. Round one to traumatised mum.

I gathered up our bags from the room, almost losing the half cucumber, and H was wheeled out to the ambulance bay. Lovely Resuscitation Nurse helped me carry and balance the bags so I could hold Pops' hand. We wouldn't make the front cover of *Refugee Times*, especially as said nurse had grabbed a pile of emergency food packs – carrier bags containing NHS sandwiches.

'Thought you could use these,' she said, conspiratorially. 'I grabbed you a couple extra, you might need them later.' We'd landed the kindness crack squad. The thought of sarnies, crisps, juice and fruit almost made it feel like we were heading off for a picnic. The mood was upbeat, as if we should have stowed lashings of ginger beer.

It took a while for the team to set up H's drip. It seemed some hook was missing from the ambulance kit. Actually, I thought a fair bit seemed missing from the ambulance, like sterile surfaces and a recent equipment check. I figured it was why there had been such a concerted effort to find a fully stocked resuscitation pack on the ward. I guess ambulances get used often. But are they always so shabby inside? What stories could this one tell?

I kept smiling at H, holding his hand, asking if he was alright, telling him how exciting it was, being in the back of an ambulance. Yes, OK, I heard my own words, couldn't quite believe them. Exciting? Being in the back of an ambulance. The pressure was clearly getting to me.

H's pallor was ghastly; how could a living person be so pale? And why does white bedding tucked around a patient look more like a shroud than anything else? He was strapped onto the trolley.

He was trying to raise a smile but it was all too much. Pops was quiet, she didn't want to let go of my hand. I settled her into the seat, which pulled down to face the top of H's trolley bed. She seemed as invisible as she needed to be on this trip. And she didn't even want a sandwich. Or juice. It must be overwhelming for her. Blimey, it was for me. How must all this make a seven-year-old feel?

'Are we all OK?' asked Bill or Ben.

'Well, apart from the cancer, we're fine' I quipped. Everyone laughed. Well, the grownups did.

We set off down the hill, away from the sea towards the M5, I tried to keep my arm across Pops' torso, keep her a bit safer. I quickly realised it was no good for my back. I'd be more use to both my children, if I could still walk by the time we got to Bristol. My daughter looked tired. She didn't once ask about blue flashing lights.

The setting sun dominated as we moved up country. I was sitting on a bench facing sideways, next to Lovely Resuscitation Nurse, who was chatty just the right amount. I looked out through the back windows of the ambulance and could see the most beautiful of sunsets developing. Deep pinks were streaked with glowing gold threads bleeding into hues of the most intense orange. Framed by the black outline of the back window seals of the ambulance, the sky was a moving picture. Such beauty; such pain. It was more surreal than a Dali or a Magritte. It was the first time any of the three of us had been in an ambulance.

Rush hour traffic coincided with the darkening sky above Bristol. Bill and Ben flicked on a satnav to try and get us round traffic queues. We ended up driving around an overgrown industrial estate, weeds pushing through tarmac. Despite the awfulness of our situation, it was quite funny. I don't really know why; guess you had to be there.

As we re-joined the main route into the city it dawned on me how much our lives were about to change. It wouldn't just be dealing with this terrible affliction that could take my son. Everything was changing. I had shunned city living for a rural lifestyle less than two years previously. We three had thrived on the moors, the beaches – or so I thought... Yet here we were, driving into the heart of a city with all its noise, pollution, people and twenty-four-hour activity.

I think that journey, in the back of a raddled old ambulance with a grounded, chatty nurse and two very kind men was the last bit of 'normal' H, Pops and I experienced for a considerable time. I was hanging onto the familiarity of that small moving space and I didn't want to let it go. Would they have to carry me out of the ambulance too?

When we arrived, as the ambulance pulled up in the bay outside the automatic front doors of Bristol Children's Hospital, it was a reality check of the highest order.

Bill, Ben and Lovely Resuscitation Nurse attended to H and trolleyed him out of the back of the ambulance and into the foyer as I grabbed bags and helped Pops. Suddenly we were again in a bright, Neon-lit space bustling with people and strangeness.

In the coming months I was to see so many people getting out of the back of ambulances in that bay. Children on trolleys, babies in incubators, swaddled toddlers clasped in the arms of a shell-shocked parent. Grey coloured grownups who looked confused, bemused, scared, drawn. That day it was me looking all those things.

The building was all glass and chrome, luminous, busy, purposeful. Not a hint of boutique hotel here, no classy piece of upholstery to offset the glass and metal, no vase of imported blooms perched artfully at reception. I smiled at my children.

'Hey H! It's a huge hospital. Much better than the last one, it's especially for children. I wonder who we'll meet. Shall we go and find some doctors?'

He tried to smile, his lips looking so big and red in his pale, shrinking face.

'Oh mum, of course we'll find some doctors.'

Through the double doors, across the lobby, past reception. I assumed Bill and Ben knew where they were going. Were they regulars on this route? By the time we got to the lifts I realised one of them was carrying one of my bags, he must have seen me struggling and stepped in so unobtrusively I hadn't even noticed. Don't cry. Don't cry. Please don't cry.

We all got in the lift, lined up by H's trolley, someone pressed a button. Out we came to clean lines, past signs, doors, corridors, lights on ceilings. Oh God, lights on ceilings. I remembered being flat on my back, on a trolley, staring up at lights on ceilings, whizzing above my head. It had, at the time, been the worst day of my life. November 1999. The day I lost a baby and had to have the 'remains' surgically removed. A year later H was born. Now, nine years on, he was on a trolley, lights on ceilings whizzing above his head.

Our peculiar little procession turned a corner and, hanging from on high, in a gap between strip lights, was an illuminated sign. Is everything in hospital illuminated? Do hospital designers believe bright lights cure illness or something?

The sight of the sign hit me so hard I thought my legs were going to buckle. There it hung, like a portent in the sky, the sign which said, 'Paediatric Oncology' and underneath, 'Ward 34'. Nothing familiar here at all. Paediatric Oncology. In your face whiteness. Stark reality. Paediatric Oncology. Clinical, no escape. Paediatric Oncology.

We were here to save H's life. I felt sick. I wanted to run. The second time I'd had that compulsion in less than twenty-four hours and I didn't even own any trainers. Now I wanted to run back to the ambulance and hide. Hide under a blanket in a corner, refuse to come out. But that really wouldn't have been very mature. Was it so very wrong to want another five minutes of 'normal'?

Doors, buttons, intercom. Antibacterial hand wash.

'We have H for you,' said Bill or Ben.

Pops and I followed H's trolley into a room, where he was gently lifted on to the bed by four people. I didn't want Bill, Ben and Lovely Resuscitation Nurse to go. At that moment they felt like the closest I had to friends in a strange new world.

I thanked them for their kindness: They knew what they had done to help us. I wished them a safe journey home. In return we were wished 'good luck' and as the room seemed to lose all its air, the three of them were gone.

I have little recollection of exactly what happened next in Room Four. With relief I spotted the pull-down bed, so I knew I Pops would be able to sleep later. The room itself was small. Even if the chair – dull turquoise plastic, of course – had been a proper recliner there was nowhere for it to recline. But there was an en-suite loo with a basin and shower, plus a white basin in the room.

A nurse checked H's temperature, pulse, blood pressure, oxygen levels. His temperature was raging. His drip was checked and another bag fitted. His cannula was fiddled with, something was run into it. Pops slumped in the turquoise non-recliner. I asked for some water. A jug with a lid – which looked NHS standard issue and in use since the 1950's - was placed on a cracked terracotta tile of the window sill. Both my children looked as uncomfortable as I felt. H was now sporting two white plastic ID bracelets, one attached to each wrist. He had gone from nine-year old boy to statistic.

'Does he have any allergies?' someone asked.

'I don't think so', I said. 'Can we have glasses for the water please?'

No one mentioned Pops. Some small, clear plastic 'glasses' arrived.

By early evening Doctor Mike - charming, good looking, an unusual twang to his accent – came to see us. He asked lots of questions and explained we would see the consultants in the morning, who would be able to tell us exactly what the blood tests had shown. Then they would be able to work out a treatment plan.

'Do you know how long we might be here?' I asked.

'Well, that depends,' he said.

I was learning fast. There are no easy answers with cancer, and leukaemia is tricky. Lumps are hard enough to predict, second guess, remove, shrink. But when cancer is in your very blood, when cancer is a liquid – well, you can see how tricky this was going to be. It's not worse, just different.

Until H's blood results had been scrutinised, my questions couldn't be answered. But I was told H was likely to have surgery tomorrow, Tuesday, so his 'wiggly' could be fitted.

A wiggly is a valve surgically implanted into the chest with a direct line into the heart and jugular vein, so chemo and other drugs could be administered swiftly and painlessly. It would also be used to take bloods and give him transfusions. The cannula in his left hand could be taken out, which I was relieved about. It was looking a bit manky. The darkening bruise seemed so big on his hand. H didn't like the cannula, he kept asking how long he would have to have it. It had already been well used.

Doctor Mike explained H would need a general anaesthetic to insert the wiggly and they would take a lumbar puncture – remove fluid from his spine – to test the state of his bone marrow. His bedside manner was straight forward; he was calm and reassuring without attempting to lessen the gravity of H's health. Here was a medic who had clearly been paying attention in the 'do not patronise parents' lectures. I appreciated that from the outset, and made it clear I was a straight-talker.

He told us to get some sleep. I mentioned the 'probable swine flu' diagnoses. Did I imagine his facial expression going from calm to OMG in about three nano seconds? He left the room very quickly, the stench of non-communication permeating the stale air.

But hey, we had some books and a bag of clean pants, half a cucumber. Our lives had hardly been a fairy tale up to then. But fairy tales don't half come in handy when your own life could have been penned by Shakespeare. And you really couldn't make this one up.

CHAPTER SIX

Activity around H felt constant. Pops was shattered. After a bite from an egg mayonnaise sandwich from emergency rations, I tucked her into bed, the pull down one, using blankets and sheets I found in the laundry cupboard up the corridor. No one said anything

Doctor Mike's parting words, *'try and get some sleep'*, left me slightly bemused. Even if I felt like it there was nowhere for me to sleep, though at one point the floor did look appealing.

H ate half a kiwi fruit, which I had been able to cut up using my trusty Swiss Army knife. Now, I don't normally carry a knife with me – or wear a hoodie, unless it's terribly chilly – but I'd been using the knife to cut dead stalks on the allotment. The allotment! Oh no!! What would happen to it now? We'd only taken it on that year and I had plans. Guess that's the end of that then.

Having my penknife gave a link to home. I had bought the small red knife – blade, corkscrew and bottle opener – for travelling in India more than twenty years ago. It had opened many a bottle, sliced much cheese and many tomatoes. It was such a happy accident to find it in my handbag. How else would I slice up the cucumber? Now we must surely be edging towards a *'ten top tips for refugees'* mini feature.

Pops slept. H lay in his hospital bed, neither asleep nor awake. By the early hours of that Tuesday morning, I felt stiff, out-of-sorts and my eyes were red raw. The institutional non-recliner was exceedingly uncomfortable and I couldn't possibly drink any more tea. I asked a very pretty nurse with short dark hair if I could use the bed in the empty room next door. Her colleague nodded. If I'd had any idea what was to follow – if the hospital had had any idea what was to follow - I would never have asked and they would never have agreed. I was feeling so grotty I had to lie down.

The ward seemed quiet. Apart from a child's voice coming from the room the other side of H's.

'It hurts mummy. I don't like it. It hurts. Take it out.' The voice seemed to be on a continuous loop.

I lay on the bed in the room next door to my children, fully dressed, under a blanket from the laundry cupboard. My head was pounding, my throat so sore it hurt to swallow, but I couldn't sleep. I kept checking on H and Pops, my mind unable to shut down. The whirring thoughts probably could have powered a small electrical sub-station.

I was worried about a bite on my foot that was full of pus. Doctor Mike had said H would be prone to every infection going. The leukaemia had wrecked his immune system and the chemo would destroy it completely. He would be vulnerable to bacteria, viruses, fungal infections - one mushroom or two?

Everything now felt threatening. What if my infected bite made him ill? Must get plasters. This was a hospital, they'd have some. I could ask. I should start writing my questions down otherwise I'd forget things. If knowledge is power, I was going to make damn sure I learnt as much as I could about leukaemia, become a powerful enemy.

The more questions popped into my head the more I realised

how ignorant I was. I knew virtually nothing about leukaemia; or chemotherapy, blood counts, thermometers you stick in ears, Bristol and Banksy. I didn't know doctors don't wear white coats any more – more likely to be a Boden skirt or Gap shirt – and I had no clue nursing staff were ranked by their colour-coded uniforms. I didn't know where I could buy a packet of Paracetamol, a packet of crisps - tampons. Until the day before yesterday I didn't even know children got cancer.

Despite my travels, a career in journalism and forty-odd years of hard living it was becoming clear I knew Jack Shit, about anything that really mattered.

I was now in a world where everyone around me – apart from my children – assumed I knew how everything worked, where things were. The three of us were in an alien environment, yet to everyone else it was a natural and familiar place. I had no sense of the hospital, no idea what floor we were on and certainly no idea what the next hour may hold, let alone the next few days.

In a few hours I would find out what shape the immediate future might take. My head hurt. Must get some Paracetamol from somewhere. I felt hot. Must be the hospital atmosphere. I kept telling myself a headache was a piffling inconvenience next to cancer.

By seven o'clock I was up and showered, unusual for me; I'm a child of the night, not of the morning. Pops was in and out of sleep. H was unchanged. I was helping him pee into a cardboard wee bottle. He was too weak to get out of bed.

Someone asked if we would stay in Room Four to see the doctors, who would explain everything. We waited. There is a lot of waiting in hospitals. Waiting to see doctors. Waiting for drugs. Waiting for blood to arrive. Waiting for information, nurses, water, scan appointments, clean sheets. Waiting for teachers, dieticians, physiotherapists, play specialists, social workers, porters, cleaners, bed pans, visitors, phone calls, parcels, letters, answers and toast.

Waiting. Waiting. Waiting. More waiting...

I didn't know all that back then. So we just waited a bit more. We no longer had somewhere to be anyway.

Someone, a nurse I think – or was it a healthcare assistant, hadn't figured the ranking colours – asked about 'the swine flu'. *Where had the diagnosis come from? When had it been given?* All three of us had to give throat and nose swabs. The throat swab was particularly unpleasant. Pops and I both gagged.

I wasn't worried. If H had had swine flu, he would be over it by now. And there seemed to be other far more important things to worry about. Surely cancer trumps swine flu?

The moment Doctor John and Doctor Michelle arrived in Room Four, along with Doctor Mike, it was like someone had hit the 'Thunderbirds Are Go' button. It was official. H had Acute Mycloid Leukaemia. He would need four intense rounds of chemotherapy. The treatment was so aggressive he might need a heart transplant. If the chemo failed, he would have to have a bone marrow transplant.

Dr Michelle – smart, expensive trousers that could have been tailored for her – said H could have anything up to twenty general anaesthetics. Well, I had asked. No one could say how many, it all depended on how he reacted to the treatment. I'd told them I wanted it straight and they had listened. Heart transplant? Bone Marrow transplant? Bloody hell. He was only nine. Oh my God – a heart transplant?

How long it would take H to get well, depended upon how sick they could make him first, how fast his body was able to recover. The plan was for the chemotherapy to take his body to the brink, four times. Each time the drug protocol was designed to destroy his immune system, blast the malformed white blood cells out of existence. Four times he would become neutropenic, a state where the body has no immune system. With no immune system a patient is vulnerable to any passing bug, vacationing virus, scrap of dirt or particle of fungus.

Dr John - tall, bespectacled possibly a bit younger than me - said we were likely to be in Bristol around six months. Six months? Oh my God, six months!

They told me it was a very aggressive form of leukaemia, more often diagnosed in those past middle age. But advances in treatments during the last twenty years meant children had a much better chance of surviving into adulthood. Survival! That word again.

The doctors explained treatment protocols were vigorous and based on knowledge shared worldwide. UK protocols were most closely aligned to those used in Finland. They would be happy to answer any questions.

By then I had a pile of questions, none of which I wanted H or Pops to hear. They agreed to meet me later, away from Room Four, which was already becoming a place of safety to scurry back to. It was also a room of fear. My mind was in overdrive.

It must take incredible professional courage to deliver such devastating news to frightened parents. I later learned Dr John had young children, Dr Michelle didn't. They subsequently both admitted they could have no idea what it was like to receive such news. I appreciated their honesty and, in particular, Dr John's dry wit. I grew to wonder if Dr Michelle had chosen her profession over a family life. It was none of my business, but it didn't stop me wondering.

I asked when H was likely to go to surgery, to have his wiggly fitted. They didn't know. Someone would check the theatre lists. Swine flu was mentioned, it felt like an aside.

As they left, I turned off the main overhead light - again. Minutes later 'a nurse' in yellow switched it back on again. Bright, glaring lights are not for me. Natural light is far more restful. H was trying to doze and Pops was sleepy. Seemed like I wouldn't even be allowed control of the light switch. It was going be a bundle of laughs that one, over the next six months. Six months! We could be in Bristol for six months. Now it wasn't the allotment which worried me – what about the cats, the house plants? What about our home???

My mobile kept ringing. Texts kept arriving. How was I supposed to know the bloody postcode? I didn't even know where the toilet up the corridor was. What floor were we on? I may as well have been in a high security prison wearing handcuffs and a blindfold.

CHAPTER SEVEN

DESPITE BEING INCARCERATED IN THIS TINY HOSPITAL ROOM, WE HAD chucked an enormous boulder into the calm of our tranquil Devon pool. The ripples tsunamied.

My second-hand mobile, formerly the ex-mother-in-law's, would have been ringing off the hook, had it had one. When it wasn't ringing it was buzzing crazily, like a toxic bee. I didn't even know who was sending some of the texts. Did I imagine the phone was feeling the strain, or was I feeling the strain? No, it was definitely playing up and for some reason wouldn't charge properly. *'Great!' I thought, 'just the right moment in life to be phoneless.'* Better than witless, I guess, although...

My pay-as-you-go had taken on its own life, dragging behind it our former life as if it was clutching a 'comfort blanket' it refused to give up. The tsunami of ripples was unstoppable. 'Man Down' – sorry – 'Boy Down'.

'Oh Sharon, we've just heard. What can we do? It must be awful. How did you find out? Where are you? And how long will you be there? How long? Will he really lose all his lovely hair?'.

On and on, call after call. You may ask yourself why I answered the phone at all, but back then I felt I had to talk to people, reassure people, play it down. It became overwhelming. I was sick of hearing my own voice repeat the same phrases over and over. It was becoming increasingly obvious H was getting worse and I didn't want to think it, let alone talk it. He couldn't get out of bed to use the toilet. He was too hot to wear pyjamas. He was becoming less responsive, spoke little and could barely drink even water.

I had to get real. I was not running a multi-million-pound business or auditioning for The Apprentice. My son was very ill, Pops was confused and looking pretty rough. I felt hideous and here I was trying to tell so many people everything was OK. But if I didn't talk to people no one would know anything. I couldn't play ostrich.

By then I was also having to bat away the numerous *'when can we come and see you?'* calls from my parents and my brother and their dad and friends, all of which were intensifying.

And then I got a call from my ex-mum-in-law, who was still in Spain.

'How are you all doing?' came the fake chirpy query from across the European airwaves.

'We're doing OK thank you. How are you doing? Is it hot? Yes, they're doing OK. Yes, see you when you get back' I said.

I knew someone had blabbed. Ex-mum-in-law is not the most subtle of beings. No one would admit to having told her. Still, good to know my family still knew better than I did. Good to know even in a crisis nothing really changes. Those closest to you are as familiar as a favourite cardi, their behaviour as ingrained as the beetroot stain on your best shirt. Thanks mum!

Still, no time to dwell, here come the next wave of calls. Or not; the phone silenced itself and chose 48 hours into our developing crisis to throw a wobbly. These devices are not inanimate objects, I simply know it.

I never realised we knew so many people. I had no idea H had made such an impression on so many people. I never knew how caring our friends were. In a quiet moment the realisation we were still part of two communities helped me to understand the response to our plight. We had moved less than two years previously from the sprawl of Reading in Berkshire to a quiet, backwater town near Exeter, Devon. In a small town, news travels fast. And people talk.

Time slowed.

I asked a nurse if there was any update on H's op, if his *wiggly* was going to be put in that day, as I had been told. No one seemed to know. I was becoming increasingly anxious, I just wanted to get things moving, blast these evil white cells out of his body, get him better. The sooner his *wiggly* was fitted, the sooner we could move on, go home. We waited for an answer. Then waited a bit more.

How many other children were on the ward, I wondered? Did the other parents feel like refuges too? How common was AML, how could I find out more? I'd been specifically told not to look on the internet, but how could I anyway? Unless there was a James Bond-style cupboard in the room, with a secret laptop concealed behind the cocktail cabinet, adjacent to the sunken bath. There wasn't even a fridge. What's the point of a cocktail cabinet with no ice? I had no appetite anyway, for food let alone a fizzing glass with a pink umbrella. We may as well have been marooned on a desert island.

Someone had promised leaflets about AML, but none arrived. I made a cup of tea in the parents' kitchen, cleaning a pile of mugs and burning my hands because the tap water was so hot. Pops and I perused a shelf of children's DVDs by the nurses' station, along the long corridor.

I felt like a lost soul yet I was having to be the life and soul, be *normal* for my children. I saw people I figured were other parents, but this wasn't a trendy coffee shop or a cinema queue, a place to idly chat. The mood was sombre, the air itself felt as if it was fighting to get out, circulate freely in an atmosphere away from the ward. It was stifling.

Word came back about the op. The doctors wanted to try and stabilise H before giving him a general anaesthetic, said Dr Mike, so they were going to delay the op until tomorrow, Wednesday. It had been a hard decision, he said. I was disappointed, I wanted to get rid of the *'crazy blood'* coursing round my son's veins. I wanted to be on the road to better, the path to well. We needed to be strolling through the gate of normal – well, as normal as any quirky creative wants to be...

I was ignorant back then. It probably made it easier. I later learnt it was a deliberate tactic, the 'drip drip' of information from on high. It's better that way, each person can take on board as much as they are able, when they are able. Some parents had little interest in the science of their child's illness. Me? I was determined to go for the PHD – knowledge is power - but I was still playing catch up. Where were those leaflets? Knowledge is power.

'Fancy a bit of cucumber?' I asked as cheerfully as I could. Pops looked at me as if I was barmy. H looked me in the eye. They both knew the cucumber was for the chop and we didn't mean thinly sliced into a lightly buttered, white bread sandwich of the genteel variety, a light sprinkling of freshly ground pepper, cut into crust-less triangles. I lobbed it in the bin marked 'non clinical waste' by the door, though by then it would have felt quite at home in a lab on a petri dish.

'Alright then H, if you could have anything you wanted right now, what would it be?' I said, meaning food.

'I want to see the cats. I want to see Oscar and Ruby. Do you think they're OK mummy?' He looked at me.

'I'm sure they'll be fine,' I said, learning to perfect the 'don't-worry-everything-will-be-fine' voice, the one I was trying hard to practice at every given opportunity. I'm sure I sounded more like a failing actress in a dying soap opera. 'Becky will feed them later,' I said.

'But they don't know where we are,' wailed Pops. 'I haven't been able to tell Ruby where we are.' Tears welled in her eyes.

'We'll talk to Becky later' I said, trying not to cry myself and wrapping her up in a hug. But I was becoming increasingly worried about the cats, very worried. If we were going to be away for six months, what on earth was I going to do about them? What about the cottage – the garden? Luckily it was a small garden and by a piece of luck I'd pruned everything right back the week before.

Our home, what would happen to our home? We had abandoned it. Our stone cottage had become a Marie Celeste tethered to the end of the M5. Washing up on the worktop, dirty washing in the linen bin, washing hanging on the radiators, fridge full, plants un-watered, carpets un-Hoovered. Our entire life had been abandoned. I wasn't complaining about Hoover abandonment ...

'Look you two,' I said, mustering all the authority I could possibly inject into a reassurance. 'The cats will be fine. I'll make sure they're looked after. But right now, it's you two I want to think about. Now let's concentrate on getting H better shall we? We're in this together – shall we see if the telly works? Apple anyone?'

In the absence of a 1970's James Bond-style cocktail cabinet I turned a cardboard sick bowl into a fruit bowl and, I'd like to think, arranged it artfully on the terracotta-tiled window sill. Eat your heart out *Changing Rooms*. Wonder if we could get Kirstie Allsop in to do a room makeover; we desperately needed a bit of vintage in here!

CHAPTER EIGHT

A tray arrived with food on it. H didn't even lift his head off the pillow. Pops glanced at the pile of beige lumps in a beige sauce, served on a bed of congealed (beige) rice, not a hint of delicately steamed Thai jasmine about it. I was already hoarding cartons of orange juice, which became apple when we realised there was actually a choice.

Nurses blurred in and out of the room. The sun set. The phone rang. Pops sought my lap and after a very long cuddle I pulled down the bed and tried to settle her in it before heading out to the parents' kitchen, to make a cup of tea.

I say 'kitchen'. It was more like a wall enclosed by a large window and a door which was more 'way' than 'door'. The space was awkward with a sink, handful of cheap cupboards, a fridge, a freezer, a kettle, a microwave and a toaster. But it also contained tea and coffee supplies. I later learnt a family had fund-raised hard to create that little kitchen, and I was dissing it ... Humble Pie.

The random mugs and assorted crockery in the cupboard were pretty rank, then my heart leapt when I spied a 'yellow Beryl' – an iconic vintage tea cup, large, which I had promptly adopted for my tea. I'd asked for vintage, and here it was, clutched in my grateful hand! Once more I was thankful I didn't drink milk. Each of the cartons I saw in the tiny fridge had names written on them in permanent black marker pen. Far too many had an abandoned, sour air about them.

The small fridge was crammed full of stuff. Half opened tubs of hummus, packets of cheese, cheese spreads, margarine, fruit, yoghurts, tubs and pots of goodness knows what. The freezer was also fairly full; lots of ready meals, microwave chips, ice cream. Nothing at all healthy looking, even the hummus tubs seemed to have a resigned air about them, as if they were guests who had overstayed their welcome by a couple of days. Another cupboard also held assorted packets of cereal, tea bags of varying sorts – some of the packets looked very dated – tins of soup, beans, opened packets of pasta. How did people cook pasta in here? But what prompted most questions was the state of the kitchen. It was unpleasant.

As I washed my chosen mug with water so hot it burnt my hands (again) I figured I may as well wash up the rest of the stuff. An attempt to do something ordinary I suppose, or simply an urge to 'do' something, clear up the cavalier attitude of other people and their dirty crockery. Still, good to see the A4 paper note Cellotaped to a cupboard door asking everyone to clear up their own stuff was effective...

I found some bleach under the sink, refusing to acknowledge the chaos inside – no, I'm not OCD, but bleach kills germs – and gave every surface a good clean, wiping it down afterwards with tear off paper stuff in a roll by the sink. Even the small table with a fold down leaf was covered in mug ring stains and melted sugar granules gluing trash mags to its chipped veneer. It wasn't quite déjà vu... But I was somewhat mystified. Surely a children's cancer ward, where infection was such an issue, should be clean? I bleached down the draining board but baulked at tackling the fridge.

As I was leaving, clutching my yellow Beryl full of steaming Earl Grey, I passed a very young woman who didn't even acknowledge my presence.

'Euwww! It stinks of bleach in 'ere,' she said to the tattooed bloke trailing behind her. 'Shove the milk in the fridge.'

Look, if you saw my roughly hewn stone cottage back in Devon, you would know I'm no *Domestic Goddess*, but that hospital kitchen was grim, particularly given its location. I suspect my old sixth form common room kitchen would have harboured less foreign bodies, and I don't mean French exchange students.

I walked the few steps back to Room 4, past the empty nurses' station, and felt once more as if I was in a parallel universe. It was either that, or a very convincing Dr Who set. We'd be running from Daleks next, but at least David Tennant would be on board. Maybe he would be able to figure which floor of the hospital we were on? Our world had shrunk to a small room with two beds, two sinks, a toilet, shower and a dodgy kitchen a few steps away, a kitchen where you couldn't even cook up a desperate bowl of pasta.

Back in the room H and Pops reproached me with their looks. "Where have you been mummy?' said Pops, accusingly. I resisted the urge to say chasing Daleks; she just wanted to be cuddled. I sat on the turquoise non-recliner and held her. She wouldn't get into the bed. All I could think was *'please let this room be clean'*.

By dark we three were beyond it and needed sleep, just to get a break from all the confusion swirling around our rather dramatic change in circumstances. My pounding head certainly needed a break. How many questions could I ask myself in 48 hours? Should I set up a mattress in the shower room for Pops to sleep on? Where could I find a mattress, just a small child's one? If

I could sort that, then at some point I could use the pull-down bed, not bother the nurses about the still empty room next door.

Pops refused to get into the pull-down bed. She wouldn't to get off my lap. When the same dark-haired nurse with the stylish pixie cut came back to check H, I asked if I could use the room next door again.

She hesitated. I was surprised. No one was in there and surely at this time of the night no one would be checked in? I still marvel at my own stupidity. But back then I had yet to be initiated into the world of childhood cancer, despite the past two days. I still saw the world through the eyes of someone who had the privacy of their own home, freedoms like popping to the shop up the road, chatting to people I knew or brewing a pot of coffee and drinking it from a clean mug out of my own cupboard. The true horror of bugs and viruses and fungus and things the wind can blow in, a person can sneeze out, what damage a drop of saliva can do, were still mysterious.

Back then I didn't know ten children a day are diagnosed with cancer and only a handful of hospitals nationwide can assess and treat them. Bristol remains the first port of call, if they have a spare bed, for any child in the South West of England – from Land's End to beyond Bath.

Childhood cancer is rare. By the time a child is diagnosed they are often very sick indeed. Too often it is an emergency, a crisis scenario because the majority of GPs are unused to seeing symptoms of cancer in children. That much I knew from our own experience. Patients can arrive in hospital any time of the day or night, in the back of an ambulance. And I was asking to sleep in one of just ten beds on the ward. No wonder the nurse had hesitated. Ignorance was not blissful but I was uninitiated and couldn't be embarrassed at that time by my request, my need, to lie on a bed.

When a second nurse came into the room and said we couldn't stay next door, I got cross.

'Well, where the hell are we supposed to sleep?' I said. 'I don't want to sleep on the floor again if there's a bed free next door. That's just daft, isn't it? Is there someone else I can ask?'

The nurses looked at each other and something passed between them. It was against all the rules, they said, but no one was due to be admitted. If they got a phone call, we would have to vacate the room - immediately.

My ire had been deflated and I thanked them both, profusely. Number two nurse had been as arsy as me, but we seemed to have reached an uneasy truce.

The dark-haired nurse was called Zoe. She must have seen our predicament far more clearly than I was able to. I also realised they were becoming increasingly concerned about H and a doctor was called. Zoe was so kind to us that night and even gave me a black bin bag to put our dirty washing in, which she whisked off to a secret washing machine. I was so grateful. H had run out of clean pyjamas within hours of arrival, and I had no idea how long my meagre supply of knickers would last.

Doctor Mike came by to check on H. I think because he was familiar to us the situation didn't seem quite so serious.

Despite a bed, and Pops asleep on the one next to me, I couldn't settle. My head was throbbing and I was unable to find answers to most of my questions. And it's hard to sleep when you are frightened. H was deteriorating. Even to a lay person like me it was clear he was gravely ill.

I must have drifted off at some point but came to, woken by a nightmare so bad I refused to let it stay in my head. I jumped off the bed and rushed into Room 4, the screams leaving my mouth before I even knew why.

There was blood everywhere. H was half hanging out of the bed, his arm dangling, the drip stand lying on the floor, an unattached tube wriggling like a worm. In the dim light it seemed as if someone had hosed the white sheets with blood and it was dripping on the floor. I grabbed H, sat him up and tried desperately to take it all in. I knew he was breathing because he kept saying over and over *'I don't want it. I don't want it. Take it away'.*

I thought he meant the cancer. Until I realised what he'd done. H had pulled out the cannula. I propped him up and went to the door, screaming for help.

'Will someone please come and help me! Help me!' It felt like I shouted it over and over. No one had told me about the help cord. No one had told me there was also an emergency button, the 'red bat phone' of paediatric oncology. I have no idea what any of the other parents may have thought. Maybe they were asleep...

After what seemed like forever – yup, the time distortion thing that plays with your mind, it really does exist – Zoe came. She swiftly took in the situation, probably not helped by my cries of 'he's pulled it out, he's pulled it out'.

By the time H was cleaned up, his sheets changed and another cannula inserted into his left hand, Room 4 was calm. I think both H and I were in shock. I was too exhausted to sleep and too frightened to leave H alone – how had I ever thought I could sleep in a room next door, leave him on his own?

I sat with him while Pops slept next door, as I had still not perfected the art of slicing myself in two. I held his hand, mopped his brow, gave him water. When he was awake, I smiled. I knew it was a stupid thing to think, but I couldn't help feeling proud of H. Helpless as he seemed, my boy had taken direct action against his situation. He was no worse off for his actions and, although it had been fairly dramatic, it reassured me about something which had been bothering me.

I had at least one answer to my myriad questions. H was definitely as up for the fight as I was.

CHAPTER NINE

By the time traffic outside our window was in full-throttle, rush hour mode, H was 'nil-by-mouth', ready for a general anaesthetic to insert his Hickman line, *wiggly*. Not that any of us were thinking food. The housekeeper, the one in daffodil yellow, had offered tea and toast but none of us was interested. Typical, offered room service and we all declined...

Bye bye cannula (!) and hello *wiggly*. I couldn't wait for *wiggly's* removal and it wasn't even in yet. Its removal would mean H was going home. First, though, a bit of waiting... Not that our room was a peaceful or restful place to sit quietly, minding our own. There were so many people coming and going I felt we'd been checked into a mobile phone shop, on a Saturday morning.

It wasn't just nurses and doctors and healthcare assistants and a cleaner and the housekeeper. A quietly spoken woman with a Scottish accent, who said she was a teacher, came in. Would H need school that day?

'Erm, school? School?? He's a bit poorly,' I mumbled.

Would H like a story from the story teller?

'Erm, well, yes he loves stories – story teller?? - but he's having an op and I don't know what time...' I mumbled.

Would H like anything from the playroom?

'Playroom?? Well, um, I'm not sure if...' I mumbled.

Another teacher popped by, had I had a chance to fill out the forms?

'Forms, I um, err? What forms? Not sure if... 'I mumbled.

A woman bearing a brown envelope wandered in. 'Your keys for CLIC House. You'll be able to get in whenever you need to. One for the outside, the other one's got your number on it.'

Before I could ask what CLIC House was one of the nurses told me the CLIC social worker would come and see us when she could.

'Social worker? But, erm, we haven't got a social worker,' I said, anger flaring. 'I've never needed one. We have never had a social worker!'

No one asked Pops if she wanted anything.

By the time even I was fed up with my mumbling, a porter arrived to take H to theatre. One of the nurses had promised to watch Pops while I was with H. No one could tell me how long theatre would take but someone – a nurse, a doctor, a maintenance man? - said I could wait outside while he was having the op. I had promised H I would be there when he woke up.

'I've had general anaesthetics before,' I said, trying to sound blasé, 'it's fine. And it's better to be asleep when they put your wiggly in and I'll be there when you wake up. It's alright love. This is all about getting you better!'

I was as convincing as I could be. My previous experiences of a general anaesthetic had both been dreadful. I was definitely having a *Father Christmas* moment. *Smile and fib, smile and fib.* There must be a whole chapter on this in the *Parents' Training Manual,* the one I have never managed to obtain a copy of...

I had my first *general* when I was five years old. Coming to after a tonsillectomy – it was the height of fashion back in 1960's and 1970's – another girl was being wheeled back from her op, screaming and covered in blood. Some idiot told me she had woken up half way through the operation.

The high-ceilinged Victorian children's ward had had a touch of the *workhouse* about it. My parents weren't allowed to visit in the three days I was there. Some boys pulled the ear off my little brown teddy and I was forced to eat soggy cornflakes for breakfast, which made me sick. My Mum had been late to pick me up and I thought I'd been abandoned, condemned to a world of shiny oblong wall tiles, blood spattered sheets and screaming children. I picked up an infection, developed an allergy to penicillin and took several weeks to recover.

My second op under general anaesthetic came thirty years later, for an ERPC – Evacuation of Retained Products of Conception – which was just as distressing as the terminology sounds. The miscarriage was bad enough, but I came round from the anaesthetic sobbing so badly the nurse had to call a doctor because she thought I was going to choke. Happily, I was awake one year later, when H was born by emergency caesarean. The anaesthetist was a right scream; at one point I was laughing so much they had to ask me to stay still so I could be stitched up.

Nine years on and I'd promised H I'd be with him all the way. By the time we got to a door on another floor (up or down, in the lift? I have no recollection) my hand was virtually Super-glued to the hospital trolley. We were led into a small anti-chamber where several gowned men stared at us.

One of them said 'Hello mum,' then turned to H.

'Hello H,' he said, 'I'll be looking after you today and I'm going to give you some 'penguin milk', to put you to sleep, while we put your *wiggly* in.'

H looked up at me and grinned. ''Penguin milk', just like Pops.' I wanted to punch the air in triumph. When Pops had her appendectomy the year before she was given 'penguin milk'. I suggested maybe H could have some for his op too (of course I'd applied the *smile and fib smile and fib* principles of parenting). Somehow it made it look as if I actually knew what I was talking about. It gave H comfort and confidence. Hurrah for 'penguin milk'!

Wonder who gets the job of milking the penguins? I mused. When the going gets tough the tough get surreal – or was I just bonkers?

H smiled and, as I held his hand, his smile grew bigger and his eyes closed. It was so fast.

One of the gowned men said, 'You can let go now mum.' It took me a while to register he was talking to me. I held on to H's hand, unable to let go.

'Come on mum,' said another one of them, 'we need to get going.'

I felt like my son was about to be abducted by a blue gown wearing cult. One of them removed my hand from H's, which by then was limp. The nurse/healthcare assistant/porter attempted to peel my other hand away from the top bar of the trolley (by then I had mentally applied the Super-glue) and I was gently edged out of the anti-chamber. Once outside I scanned the corridor for chairs.

'They said I could wait outside,' I almost shouted at the young woman. 'They said I could wait outside while he was in theatre and there aren't any chairs. Where are the chairs?'

Somewhat bemused the young woman looked at me.

'No one waits outside theatre,' she said, ever so gently. 'Come on, let's get you back to the ward.'

'But they said I could. I told H I would be here, waiting for him,' and I promptly burst into tears, turned away from her obvious concern and balled my fists into my eyes, feeling like a right plonker, trying to stem the flow. It felt like someone had turned on a tap and unwound the garden hose. I needed a table-cloth for a hankie. Or a hug.

'It's OK,' she said, 'they'll tell us as soon as he's coming round and I'll bring you back. This happens to lots of parents, it's all very emotional.'

Get a grip said a mumble inside my head. And say *thank you*. She's being kind and she's so young, she's really got no idea. It's not fair to take out your feelings on her.

I complied, followed her back to the ward (lift? Stairs? Up? Down? I don't remember) all the while seething because someone had so blatantly lied to me. It was a lie; a downright lie and they must have known all along no one waited outside theatre. I had wanted to be close to H, that's all. Somehow the thought of being just a few meters away, just a couple of walls between us, had made it easier to deal with, easier to think I could help, 'will' him through it.

Yet I was forgetting something quite fundamental. Having been inducted into the grand world of hypocrisy when I became a mother, where the 'rules' say you must bring up your child to be honest and tell the truth (well, in my world, anyway) you spend much of your time lying to them. And now here I was, back in the land of *Father Christmas* where we expect children to actually believe the big man in red comes down the chimney once a year (stop it!) and delivers the presents his elves have been making all year to the *good* children.

I was now in the world of the great unknown, a place where no one, not even the most experienced of paediatric oncologists, could tell me what was actually going to happen. I was in the land of *Father Christmas* – with the *Easter Bunny* and the *Tooth Fairy* thrown in for good measure. We were ensconced in a world where there would be questions with no answers, scenarios with no outcomes, days without a beginning or an end. Some people would placate me because it was easier. '*Yes of course you can wait outside theatre*' was easier than telling me I couldn't.

For a woman whose favourite word is '*why?*', I already knew this was going to be a tough experience. I'm much better with people who are able to admit *'I don't know'* rather than those who resort to bullshit.

My tears had dried. My resolve that all three of us would survive H's cancer meant throwing all the bloody mince pies and tinsel out the window. The rush of adrenaline made me feel physically sick but the sight of Pops sitting on her own, back in the hospital room, brought tears back. As I held her on my lap, I couldn't believe I had opted to sit outside theatre while H was unconscious, leaving Pops on her own. How the hell was I going to find a way to care for both my children in the coming weeks – months?

'One day at a time' is how. The mumble was not just a sound in my head, it was talking sense.

On this day, however, it was one hour at a time. No one had been specific as to how long H would be in theatre, but I was told it was a straight forward procedure, it wouldn't be *'too long'*.

'Someone will come and get you when they've finished,' said a nurse/healthcare assistant/porter.

'I promised him I'd be there when he came round,' I said, 'I need to be there when he's in recovery.'

The 'whoever' repeated HER mantra. 'Someone will come and get you when they're ready.'

'I promised him,' I said, 'I promised him I'd be there. Do they ring down or send someone?'

She smiled at me, nodded and walked off. I couldn't blame her. My emotion was one of fear, born of experience. Here was a nurse used to dealing with parents in many states of angst.

Pops and I waited. And of course, when you need a distraction, you're not going to get one.

No one came into the room, so we went for a wander. We found the playroom, by walking past the parents' kitchen. It was geared up for young children with dolls and a pram and ride on stuff and games and locked cupboards. Locked cupboards? No one was there and Pops didn't feel like playing any more than I felt like hitting the *play-mode* button, which meant engaging the *jolly* segment of my brain.

We went back to Room 4, on the way looking at the shelf stacked with DVDs. An older woman, wearing a top designed to blend into the background, was sat at the end of the nurses' station, inputting data onto a large screen.

She must have seen us looking at the shelf and assured us we could borrow them, that they were there to be borrowed. Pops chose some she thought H would like and we took them back to the room. Thank God she chose more than one!

After about an hour I began to ask nurses about H. When they were either getting pissed off with me, or concerned it had been quite a while, someone called theatre. No news.

Ten minutes later: Still no news. I was beside myself yet trying to stay calm for Pops. This wasn't right. This wasn't right at all. He was having a *wiggly* fitted and a bone marrow sample taken from his spine. Both were straight forward procedures – I had been told – and should not be taking this long.

I left Pops in Room 4 and went looking for answers. Uncomfortable looks from nurses were not helping. Was I turning into the mother from hell? Probably. But I didn't care. I wanted to know H was alright. I needed to know H was alright.

After what had been far too long I was escorted – well, led actually, I was still terribly disorientated – to theatre recovery. As I walked in through the door, I knew my instincts had been spot on. H was NOT alright.

I shot across the room to his bed on the left-hand wall, furious he was awake and I hadn't been there, the fury spent as I registered there was a nurse and an older man in scrubs both trying to hold H down and place a mask over his face. Instinctively I went to the empty side of the bed, held H's hand and started talking, getting as close to his ear as I could.

'It's OK H, mummy's here. I'm here, it's OK. I'm here. H. H, it's OK.' Almost immediately there was a calming in H's demeanour. But his thrashing didn't stop.

'What on earth has happened?' I said, the words spilling out so fast I must have sounded as if I was on something. Looks were exchanged between nurse and scrubs man.

It transpired there had been *complications*. The procedure had not been straight forward. 'Something happened in theatre', said one of them. H's oxygen levels had dropped very significantly. With a serious lack of healthy red blood cells carrying even less oxygen around his body, it was essential to get his levels up. The pair were trying to put a large mask over his face, to get the oxygen from the cylinder by the trolley into his lungs. And he didn't like it. Not sure I would have either, coming round from a drug induced sleep to find two complete strangers trying to force a big plastic thing over my face.

'What do you mean 'something happened?'' I said, soon realising taking it out on these two wouldn't help H.

'We have to get him to breathe what's coming out of the mask,' said tall, scrubbed man, 'but he won't let us put it over his face.'

Hoping my look wasn't too withering I said I'd have a go. Would it be OK if I held it over his mouth and nose rather than holding it down?

'Give it a go,' said Mr Scrubs, 'get him to breathe.' The nurse watched the monitor H was hooked up to, avidly.

I don't know how long we were in recovery, until H calmed down and his oxygen levels rose enough so Mr Scrubs was prepared to release him back to the ward. At one point I'd asked for some ice, or even better an ice pop. I figured while he was sucking on something his breathing would calm – an old trick from my own experiences. To the surprise of the nurse, she found one from somewhere close by. Why on earth was she surprised?

Were the regulars off sick? Was she in training, drafted in from a bunion ward?

The only explanation I ever got for what happened in theatre was that one of H's lungs had *probably* collapsed during surgery. No one was ever able to tell me *why*. The most important thing was that H got out alive, with his *wiggly* in place. How many more dramas could any of us could cope with? How much living could any one person pack into just three days?

As it turned out, rather a lot.

CHAPTER TEN

Pops' eyes bulged at the state of her brother being wheeled back into Room 4, his face covered by an over large plastic mask, hooked up to a canister of oxygen.

The atmosphere in the room had changed significantly. The *click click click* of the oxygen machine felt so loud. It was as if each laboured breath made its presence felt, deepening the knowledge his diseased blood, silently circulating, was dragging him further away from us. It may sound overly dramatic, but it was terrifying witnessing how fast H was declining. The fear of those three little words, *forty per cent,* was intense.

Dr Mike came into the room. He was clearly concerned. So was the other doctor, her long black hair contrasting with the white coat she had chosen to wear, her accent aligned with the colour of her Asian skin.

All Pops and I could do was sit in the room, be there with H. I noticed a family had been checked in to the room next to us, Room 5. It would be the floor for me. I filched some extra sheets and blankets from the laundry room I'd found up the corridor.

It got dark. Apart from answering my mobile, Pops and I sat; time seemed little more than an abstract concept.

A new nurse came in, checked H's vitals.

'You'll be off to CLIC House soon then?' she said.

'CLIC House?' I said, blankly.

'Yes, CLIC House, where you're staying. It's meant to be lovely up there,' she said.

'I don't know what CLIC House is,' I said. 'We're not really staying anywhere at the moment. We only got here the day before yesterday so I don't really know what's happening yet. We were in the room next door last night.'

She gave me a funny look and repeated we'd have to get off soon. I had no idea what she meant.

'I can't leave my son,' I said, 'he's really poorly. I can't leave him.'

'Well, you've got the keys for CLIC,' she said, and was gone.

Was this the moment where you choose to laugh or cry? I did both. It was a confusing time! Had I got that right? A nurse who I'd never met before told me I had to leave the room, leave H, go somewhere else. The brown envelope! Where had I put it? That must be what she was talking about!

Pops was looking shattered and said she was cold. I wrapped her in a blanket and sat her on the turquoise chair while I found the A5 envelope. Inside were some wonkily photocopied A4 sheets with an address for somewhere called CLIC House, some 'guidelines' about things like laundry, being respectful to others, using the kitchens and two keys, one with a number on it the other marked *Front D*oor. I was getting more and more confused. But washing machines, that was good!

The new nurse came back into the room. 'Excuse me,' I said, 'can you tell me what CLIC House is please?'

She looked at me as if I was a lunatic. 'It's where you're staying,' she said, her tone of voice more suited to a small child.

'Erm. Staying? We're not actually staying anywhere,' I said, trying not to speak to her as if she was an idiot.

'Yes you are, you're staying at CLIC House', she said. 'You can't both stay here.'

'Where is CLIC House?' I said, trying to elicit something useful out of this mindless exchange.

'It's where all the parents stay. It's up the hill behind the hospital.'

'Look,' I said, attempting to appeal to her helpful, understanding, caring side. 'We arrived here on Monday evening in the back of an ambulance. I've never been to Bristol before. What hill? I haven't been any further than the playroom since we got here. I don't know what CLIC House is. I don't even know if I can afford to stay there.'

Her compassion by-pass surgery had clearly been a huge success.

'It's not that far to walk. Or you can get a taxi,' she said and bustled out of the room.

I will never know who was more mystified by the exchange; her or me, but I formed a plan. Find a taxi number. Get a lift to the mythical CLIC House. Take our bags, drop them off and then come straight back to H. That way at least I would have done what I thought I had been asked of me. I also figured it was approaching shift change and she'd be gone soon. I put Pops in her coat. Next time New Nurse came in the room it looked as if we were off. What a great ruse, wish I'd actually thought of it instead of it happening by default!

Pops and I didn't make it to CLIC House, until the following year.

New Nurse went off duty and then there was Zoe. Lovely Zoe. Zoe who immediately clocked H wasn't faring too well.

Zoe calmly told me she was going to call the doctor. She saw Pops wearing her coat. 'We can't go to CLIC House now,' I said. 'But I'll have to put Pops to bed. That other nurse said we had to go but I can't leave H. Zoe, I can't leave him.'

'Put Pops to bed,' said Zoe firmly.

'But I don't want to get you into trouble,' I said, fighting tears. 'I can't leave him.'

'No, you can't,' said Zoe. And she was gone.

I pulled down the bed and made it up for Pops. A request earlier in the day for some Calpol had not been heard. She'd had a temperature but they could only administer it to patients. How ironic. H was awash with the stuff but Pops wasn't allowed any.

I'd also asked the white coated doctor earlier if I could get some Paracetamol, for my own head. Her response had been to suggest I wait till about 11 o'clock, pop next door to the BRI A&E – when it would be quiet – and ask for some there. I had been quite stunned by her response. She could have told me where the nearest shop was! Besides, I had no idea what the BRI was (Bristol Royal Infirmary), or what 'next door' actually meant. Maybe it was 'next door up a hill'? I craved a parallel universe, much easier than attempting to try and navigate the one we were actually living in. The one in which I felt a stranger. Bring on the Daleks please. And David Tennant, of course. Can you tell we're fans?

Talking of *doctors* there seemed to be an awful lot in the room, milling in and out. Night blurred into day. Pops slept; H fought the mask until Zoe found a smaller one. It transpired H was wearing an oxygen mask designed for an adult. No wonder it had been so ineffective. Still, his oxygen levels were not going down; he seemed more stable. The oxygen click click clicked ...

I drifted through the dark hours, unable to sleep, though my mind must have periodically shut down. My head hurt with questions. My head hurt a lot. I was trying to be logical, find solutions. There were so many question marks. I wrote more lists.

I came to, on the floor by H's bed, at an ungodly hour when my phone rang. A friend offering help. I resisted the urge to say it would have been helpful if she hadn't woken us all up... I am so not a *morning person*! Still, on with the day. My whole body felt stiff, I was freezing cold despite the blankets and my head pounded, lights flashed. I was the orange flashing light on a pole sticking up from the airport luggage trolleys surrounded by the noise of jet engines from parking planes, not a sound-proofed ear muff in sight.

Pops went back to sleep. H seemed surgically attached to his bed. He was too weak to sit up let alone go to the toilet. Figuring how to help him to the loo, while attached by tubes to a drip and a machine, was a challenge too far. I held yet another cardboard wee bottle for him and took it to the sluice room, past the parents' kitchen, stocking up with some more cardboard essentials on the way back. I made tea and waited for doctors' rounds. Today they planned to start the chemotherapy. Oh God! I still hadn't told H he would lose all his hair.

A posse of doctors appeared. What is the collective term for doctors? A Dirge of doctors? A death of doctors? Certainly not a dearth. I think there were five at this point. Doctor John, Doctor Michelle, Doctor Mike and White Coat, who I think was on attachment, plus someone else I didn't know. Rather like a wolf sniffs the breeze or a tracker smells pooh, I could tell the air had changed. And the weirdest thing – they were all wearing paper masks...

Did someone take a deep breath? Was it Doctor John who spoke?

'We have the results from your swabs,' said someone.

It took me a moment to register what he was talking about before the penny didn't so much drop as come crashing through an entire skyscraper worth of reinforced glass.

'All three of you have tested positive for swine flu.'

At this point I gave probably the most inappropriate response humanly possible.

'You're joking!?' I said.

While it explained an awful lot, it was still a shock. All I could think were the words *underlying health condition*. Every swine flu death reported in the media – and by that time there were hundreds – was reported in conjunction with *'an underlying health condition'*.

There was no denying leukaemia qualified.

We were now the embodiment of every horror headline the press had been pumping out for weeks. The talk was of epidemics, rising death rates, impending apocalypse. We'd gone from swine flu to cancer in three days. Without shaking off the swine flu. I was struggling to take it all in.

I was in the middle of a doctors' convention, a train crash, a sci fi movie all at the same time. Where's the hunky lead male when you most need him? No one could say how long H had been affected by the H1N1 virus, or how long it would linger. We had probably caught it off him.

The vibe was no longer *'calm and capable'*. It was no longer *'we've been here before and we know how this may play out'*. It was *'what do we do next?'*.

There was me thinking we'd entered a living nightmare. Now it was hell on earth. A new hell on earth, never before encountered. By anyone in the known universe. Anywhere. Ever. Some people spend a lifetime looking for ways to be unique, different, special. We'd hit the jackpot, without even trying.

As the discussions continued – and I was relieved to have been included at that stage – it became very, very apparent our presence on Ward 34 was a danger to other patients. The crashing penny of the skyscraper became a Tornado jet with no pilot, set on a collision course for Room 4, primed to cause as much destruction as possible.

H was too ill to be moved. But where could they move him to anyway? If he was moved to another room, on another floor, he would not have access to the specialised medical care on Ward 34, knowledge essential for his survival. There was no way they could move him to PICU – the Paediatric Intensive Care Unit. It was too dangerous for other seriously ill children. He was too ill to be moved to another hospital where he could be treated – where he would also be a danger to other very sick children. The decision was taken to contain the problem – contain the swine flu.

Everyone who came into Room 4 had to wear a surgical mask, latex gloves and a plastic apron. Each mask, apron and pair of gloves had to be removed after each wearing. A bin for the purpose was wheeled in, a reel of plastic aprons was placed in a clanky metal container just outside our door, like a giant roll of cling film, wrapping up human beings. Even if the mask and aprons and gloves had only been worn for a few seconds they had to be binned. The bin filled up very rapidly.

No one was allowed to leave the room wearing the get up, to eliminate any chance of contamination. I was told Pops and I were not allowed to leave the room – not even to get drinking water. No more parents' kitchen. No playroom. No cups of tea. No corridor walks. No DVD choosing. No access to anything outside our very immediate surroundings.

We had become the epicentre of the sci-fi movie of my imaginings. We could no longer see the faces of the strangers who surrounded us. It felt sinister, unreal, threatening. And there was no maverick scientist charged with saving the world, no added 'love interest', no make-up artist, no script, no director shouting 'cut' before the lunch van served up.

It was just H, Pops and me in a small room with nothing but fear, uncertainty, confusion, an empty water jug and, oh yes, leukaemia.

Was it possible to become any more isolated? Could we be removed any further from our previous life? The one where I play the insignificant single mum bringing up two children in a tiny stone cottage in rural Devon, Dartmoor and the beaches our back garden? No hero in that one either. I could so use a hug.

Now everyone coming into the room – and there were so many – was a stranger, even the ones we had met. All you could see were their eyes.

What an interesting study we would make for a psychology student. A thesis, possibly: 'The Effects of Sudden and Enforced Isolation Upon a Lone Adult Nuclear Family Unit, Acclimatised to the freedom of Devonshire, Now Imprisoned in one Small Room'. Catchy, huh?

No one was joining up the dots of our life, our reality, our situation. Not one person asked where 'dad' was – maybe that was too 'un-PC'? No one said, 'you need to call someone'. And I wasn't wearing a funky badge proclaiming: 'Single Mum. Coping Alone'. Maybe people thought 'my other half' had popped out for a coffee?

By that stage all I could do was focus on functioning. Being in the room (had nowhere else to go anyway), being a positive presence for my children. Pops was poorly and clingy, H was off the scale and now I knew why I had been feeling so bloody awful. It wasn't shock or lack of sleep. It was swine flu.

Still, at least I didn't have cancer. H was now fighting swine flu AND cancer. With virtually no immune system. *Underlying health condition.* What about the chemo? *Forty per cent.*

H became the focus of intense medical activity. His drip stand was in constant use, drugs and fluids being pumped into his emaciated body. At one point they needed two drip stands. They were fighting his raging temperature with Paracetamol intravenously, by a syringe driver, which was mechanically pumping drugs straight into his body, via his *wiggly.*

A nurse called Rachel checked H's vitals. She seemed friendly, had strawberry blond hair. Apparently 'they' (the hospital pixies?) were trying to contact a social worker 'they' thought was called Arthur. Maybe he could help us?

By then I couldn't get cross about someone telling me I

needed a social worker. I needed back up. Fast. Maybe he could authorise a child's mattress, so I could setup a bed for Pops in the shower room. At least then she could get some sleep.

Nurse Rachel said the CLIC social worker would be coming to see us soon, she would be able to help. I had begun to figure CLIC was some kind of charity, helping people like us. I asked if they had any information on AML I could have.

'Don't look on the internet,' said Nurse Rachel, through her mask. 'We always advise our parents not to look it up, there's too much information out there and it can be very confusing. I'll find you a booklet.'

'Internet? Can you get the internet in here?' I said, thinking how useful that would be.

'Oh yes,' she said, 'there's a computer in a little room near the parents' kitchen. It usually works. I think. Oh, hang on. You won't be able to use it though. You have to stay in here. But Jamie will come and see you soon, he can explain everything. You'll be able to ask him anything you want.'

So, there were people out there who could help us! Jamie? Arthur? A CLIC social worker? But we needed help now, not tomorrow or next week or when someone came back from holiday. Wasn't there a matron on this ward, someone whose job it was to make sure she knew all about her patients? Maybe she was on holiday. Maybe that was why no one seemed to realise the three of us had no safety net.

Our lives had been so precariously balanced for so many years it was *normal* for me to have to cope alone; circumstance had dictated it. We had wonderful friends. Our family had their own lives.

My mum and dad lived in Dorset; my dad was not well. My ex-mum-in-law was sole carer for her older, second husband. My brother was a full-time stress cadet, when not running his own business, had a single mum girlfriend, who worked

H and Pops' dad, my ex-husband, worked full time. Each of us knew he could not have cared for both his children. He'd never had to, never wanted the role. We had separated three weeks before Pops was born. There was still a court order in place barring him from having the children on his own. Nothing sinister, a hangover from the divorce proceedings and he'd never wanted custody. He lived almost 200 miles away from our Devon cottage.

You get the picture. Geographically we are not a close family, practically we are far away. Our bonds are tied in blood lines, not shared experiences. For the three of us this was all we had known as our family unit. Here in 21st century England family structures are probably looser than they have ever been. We share our situation with an awful lot of families.

All of this may sound like a car crash life. It wasn't. It was our *normal.* Up and down the country there are countless mums – and a few dads – bringing up children alone, while working. (Gingerbread, the lone parent charity, says 95 per cent of single-parents are women). Some get every other weekend off, some don't. I don't. Some choose social lives if they have, or can afford, babysitters. Many of us have no choice. Money is tight and time is tighter. Exhaustion you learn to deal with, crap telly and books become antidotes to un-lived, silent lives. Sewing helps me. You drink lots of cold tea, wine whenever you can – or is that just me?

For H, Pops and I being together, a unit, a threesome was how we lived. What wasn't *normal* was being imprisoned in a small room. With no drinking water. And leukaemia.

I asked a masked nurse for a jug of water. She must have forgotten. I asked another one. No jug came. Just more doctors wearing surgical masks. I asked a doctor for some water. It was a bit of an 'Oliver' moment.

Please Sir, can I have some water...

CHAPTER ELEVEN

A TRAY OF FOOD ARRIVED. I PROMPTLY PLACED IT BY THE OUTER DOOR OF Room 4, where it joined several wee bottles, a cardboard pooh receptacle – delicately covered by a green paper towel which gave a gentle waft each time someone came or went. The bin of used masks, aprons and gloves overflowed while a pile of dirty bedding was also competing for space. I'm sure room service in prison would have been better. If not, we'd have heard the newspaper headlines screaming, wouldn't we?

The phone rang. I tried to charge it again, keep it going a bit longer. If the phone stopped working, we would have no connection with the outside world at all.

Mum asked when they could come and visit. The docs said visitors were not a good idea. It was hard explaining to people how much of a risk they posed to H. It was new territory for all of us. We may as well have been aboard the Star Ship Enterprise; we were slipping away from our own universe so fast and there was no 'Scotty' to fix the boosters so we could get back.

I was worried about running out of credit on my pay as you go, so when mum said she felt helpless, didn't know how to help, I asked her to top up the phone.

'It's quite simple mum, you can do it at a cashpoint,' I said.

'What, any cashpoint? It doesn't have to be a special one?' she said.

'Yes, it's pretty standard these days,' I said, while trying to get H to take a sip of water.

'I just put my card in?'

'Yes mum, as if you were getting out cash. Choose the 'top up' option, it'll come up on the screen. The instructions will guide you through, it's quite straight forward. But make sure you have my mobile number written on a piece of paper, you need to tap that in.'

'But what do I do with your phone number then? I'll already have used my pin number so why do I need your mobile number?' said mum.

'You need my number so they can top up my phone. It makes it very clear when you have to put the number in. And they ask you for it twice, to make sure it's OK. Much easier to have it written down than have to fiddle with your phone,' I said.

'When exactly do I put your number in?'

'Just follow the instructions, it's very clear,' I said, trying to be patient.

'And then what happens?'

'It's really easy mum, even I can do it!' I tried to lighten the moment.

'Yes, but I'm a pensioner and I don't know how all these things work. It's alright for your generation you were brought up on computers,' she said.

'Well, actually it was calculators in my day.' I tried to laugh but it probably sounded like someone unblocking a drain. 'Mum, it's quite straightforward,' I said, trying to speed things up. I was losing vital credit trying to explain to my mum how to put more credit on my phone.

'How much do you want?' she said.

'Whatever you want to put on would be great, thanks mum.'

Meanwhile, back in the world of hospital, talk turned to Tamiflu. The docs wanted to clear up my swine flu as swiftly as possible. They feared there was a chance H could become re-infected – from me and Pops. By God this swine flu was a rule breaker – or was it the leukaemia? I knew I could live through any side effect thrown at me – *here, cut off my arm in exchange for a healthy H, no, no, go on, it's fine, honestly!* But I didn't want Pops getting sicker. No one was sure how Tamiflu could affect a seven-year-old, but it was felt she could suffer significantly more than an adult. I went for the fifty/fifty option. I took it, in the hopes it would clear up my swine flu 24 hours quicker and you never knew when that 24 hours would come in handy. I decided Pops would not take it and the doctors were content with that.

I was a bit confused by the whole H1N1 crisis. Newspaper reports had suggested it was a horrific flu and we'd heard tell of folk in our own town who'd had it before we landed in Bristol. The urban myth had grown on the very pavements we had, until recently, trod.

'He was so ill,' someone had told me, *'they thought they'd have to hospitalise him. Then his children got it, all three of them went down. They had to quarantine the whole house. I don't know how his wife coped. It was dreadful. It's going to take him weeks to recover from it.'*

I knew hundreds had died. I knew it was bad. I knew H was desperately ill. Pops and I were ill but I'd had flu once before – proper full-blown flu, not a bad cold. I had driven home from work, collapsed into bed and was unable to move for three days.

I felt dreadful here in this Bristol 'prison' room, but I was still functioning. I had no bed to lie in and no Paracetamol to swallow. Pops was curled up under blankets and someone did eventually, at my request, give her some Calpol. Maybe for me it was the adrenalin. Or maybe it was the fear. Whatever it was, I was grateful for it. Though it felt like I was attempting to climb Everest in a pair of summer pyjamas.

I wondered how the swine flu statistics were being collated. The deaths could be attributed to swine flu because the post mortems will have confirmed the cause. But how many people had swine flu anecdotally? How much self-prescribing was going on and how many sick days were lost to hypochondriacs and fakers? If people were not routinely tested –and they weren't, logistically that was impossible – how could anyone know how far reaching H1N1 had become – could become?

H had been diagnosed at our GP surgery back in Devon as having *probable swine flu.* It had only officially become swine flu because he had been tested in a high dependency paediatric oncology ward. While I was terrified for him, I was relieved for everyone else. If I hadn't mentioned swine flu there would have been no test and no result and we would have put everyone on the ward at even more risk. If Pops and I had gone to CLIC House last night, how far could we have spread the infection? How many more families would have been affected?

Studies later showed from June to April 2010* 474 people died of swine flu, many of them young children, the pregnant or those with *underlying health conditions.* From September 2010 to May 2011 a further 563 people died, with a further 91 cases being investigated as to whether H1N1 had killed them.

It was not hard to see why swine flu hysteria had spread so quickly. We were at the epicentre of an international drama and it was no longer simply *my nine-year old son has cancer.*

Layer by layer we were being peeled away from everything familiar. If we were convicted prisoners, we'd have had less isolation, more *Human Rights.*

We had no Arthur. No Jamie. No CLIC social worker. Were they real people, or hospital myths? We had no visitors. No training manual. No significant – or insignificant - other. No water. Damn that raging thirst.

Please may I have some more water, I asked a masked nurse, who said she was called Rachel but she wasn't because Nurse Rachel had strawberry blond hair and this nurse was blond. I'd lost my home, my car, my life but I sure as hell wasn't going to lose either of my children so I'd better make sure I didn't lose my marbles as well. Two Nurse Rachels! That's it. Nurse Rachel and Nurse Rachael.

Neither could tell me when H's chemo would start. I was oblivious to most of the high-level discussions taking place in other parts of the hospital. It was not hard to work out our unfolding drama – or *Perfect Storm* as one consultant described it – was becoming a nightmare for the hospital authorities. Where's George Clooney when you need him?

CHAPTER TWELVE

THERE HAD STILL NOT BEEN A DECISION ABOUT STARTING H'S CHEMO. I wanted to get going with it. Surely, we had to fight the leukaemia as fast as possible? We were less than 72 hours into our Bristol experience, but I felt the cancer was being given free rein to cause as much havoc as it wanted. And no one was doing anything about it.

I knew the swine flu was a pretty big setback. I had no concept how much our experience to date represented gentle ripples on quarry water; the boulder was on its way.

I'd been given a booklet nattily entitled *Childhood Acute Myeloid Leukaemia (AML)*. It was time to get reading. With no access to the internet – someone had said I could plug my laptop in somewhere but not finding the plug was irrelevant, I had no laptop. The 32 pages of clinical booklet was all I had.

AML most commonly affects white blood cell production in the bone marrow and is most common in adults, rare until the age of forty, I discovered. The cause(s) are unknown, though high levels of radiation such as those experienced after the atom bomb explosions in 1945 Japan, is linked. Certain chemical exposures can increase the risk of AML, for example other chemo regimes for a previously diagnosed cancer. Benzene in cigarette smoke can be a significant factor in adult AML, Down's syndrome has been linked and familial AML has been known.

The reason for H's AML remains a mystery, there is not a direct link, uncovered by any clinical research, highlighting a common cause. Cancer doesn't necessarily need a reason to manifest, often it just does. Thankfully it is rare in the very young.

Of course, I blamed myself entirely. I was a social smoker for eleven years, gave up five years before getting pregnant the first time. I had driven out to the Ukraine in a seven-and-a-half-ton truck to deliver aid to victims of Chernobyl; we'd lived in Reading near the most polluted junction in Europe; we'd lived ten miles from AWE Aldermaston (Atomic Weapons Establishment); an aunt by marriage had died of AML in her early forties; I'd had an uncle with Down's, back in the days when they were called *Mongols,* and there is a genetic link between ALL (Acute Lymphoblastic Leukaemia) and Downs.

In reality H's AML was an irony. I avoided chemicals. At home we ate organics whenever I could afford it. When I did clean the cottage, I preferred 'green' products or vinegar to harsh chemicals and our toiletries were free of unnecessary additives wherever possible.

H's symptoms had been atypical. While he had been pale and tired, he'd had no bleeding, bruising or breathlessness and his slight, variable temperatures had been put down to the swine flu. The first warning was the pain in his leg half way up the stairs, less than four days ago. Was it really just four days since our life was stolen away? Only four days! It felt like we'd lived four incarnations in that time. I'd like to come back as a spoilt Princess living in a palace please. Oh alright, I'd probably last the weekend, unless of course it had its own private spa...

There is no skin rash with AML, though there may be bleeding gums. It takes an average of six weeks from the first symptoms to clinical diagnosis, which can only be confirmed in a lab. H had been tired and pale for some weeks.

OMG! Several weeks. To fulfil a promise, I'd saved hard for a half term trip to Disneyland Paris. It would explain why we had to keep stopping in the parks because H kept saying *'I'm a bit tired Mum, can we stop here.'*

The three of us had spent a lot of time sitting on benches. H had often not eaten, which was so unusual it had been a worry. I figured he'd had a bug, which had lowered his immune system enough to let the swine flu in. I should have acted sooner! I should have taken him to our GP more quickly. It was all my fault. It was my fault he was so ill. I looked at Disney photographs - how could I have not seen he was so pale?

I was in quite a state by the time I got to page 9 of said booklet '*Without effective treatment, AML can rapidly cause death*'. If H died it would all be my fault. *'Treatment normally starts within a few days following diagnosis'.*

My head was screaming *'start the bloody chemo today, get going'* but despite *a degree of urgency*, said the booklet, information has to be gathered so the appropriate treatment is given.

'Children may have little or no time at home, because they will usually need supportive care between courses (of chemotherapy), *but this will vary. The necessary level of supportive care can only be provided in hospital. It will include barrier-nursing to protect against infection and intensive treatment with intra-venous antibiotics or antifungal drugs if infection occurs'.*

I knew about H's *wiggly*; I had no idea about the *'special requirements for care of the child's central venous line'.* Was I supposed to be doing something? Nursing had never been a career option. The smell of sick makes me feel sick.

In some instances a child may find it difficult to eat or drink because of the side-effects of chemotherapy. In this case it may be necessary for nutrition to be given by tube ...' I just wanted to cry.

By the time phrases were jumping out at me like rogue fireworks I was sat on the toilet with the door locked so the children couldn't see me sobbing. Phrases like *'good long term survival'; 'very aggressive drug treatment'; 'results are continually being improved, especially with better control of infection'; 'likelihood of a good long-term outcome'; 'failure to achieve remission'.*

There was me thinking the last four days had been tough. I had to face this terminology. I had to learn AML inside out. H and Pops needed me and they needed me in the room, not locked in the toilet sobbing. Maybe it was hormonal. Memo to self: Must get some tampons - sharpish!

With a washed face and only marginally blotchy it was time to come out of the bathroom.

'Are you OK mum?' asked H.

How humbling is that?

With renewed determination it was time to wise up, tell the blob of wobbly jelly lurking inside my bulky frame to bugger off. If I could be positive, remain calm and look as if I was in control then it would be the best thing I could do for H and Pops. There was only one outcome I could possibly contemplate, taking both my children home. Setting goals works. We three would be home, I decided, before Pops' eighth birthday. Six months away.

I would sleep on the floor for six months if it meant getting H well, of course I could. We'd find ways of coping, things to make and do. We were a creative lot. Books to read, films to watch, medicines to administer.

The phone rang. 'Sharon, it's Chris. How you doing?'

'You've heard about the swine flu then?' was all I could say.

'Not having much luck, are you? I'm on my way, should be with you soon!'

'What do you mean? But, but, it's not really a...'

'I knew you'd say that. I just got in the car. I had to come. I'm about half an hour away, see you soon, bye.' And the phone went dead.

About half an hour later a woman wearing a ridiculous skirt, lots of purple and hair so curly bonkers it had to be tied down, walked into Room 4. Even wearing a surgical mask, I could tell she was grinning through tears.

CHAPTER
THIRTEEN

It was hard not cry at the sight of Chris. Her plastic apron crinkled as we hugged. H raised a half smile.

Like so many, Chris had heard about our plight with increasing horror and, feeling helpless, had taken matters into her own hands. It's one of the reasons why we have always got on. There is something very powerful about a friend who drops all her own stuff and comes charging in to help, unasked.

I knew she'd have had to rearrange a shed-load of happenings just to come and see us. Words tumbled out of both our mouths. The relief of seeing a friendly face – well, pair of eyes! – was overwhelming and caused a wave of emotion so huge I had to sit down. It was like being knocked off your feet by an enormous Cornish wave. Both of us were gabbling so much it probably looked like we'd swallowed a bucket of sea water.

Another reason why I like Chris is because she often knows what needs doing before anyone has said anything. Her uber-organisation can be scary and is off-putting to some people. But if you're trapped in a small hospital room with a very sick child, a poorly child, no route to the outside world and you're in a state of shock, then she's the woman for the job.

Chris and I met because we'd had two things in common, at the same time. Very young sons and a fabric-crazed love of patchwork and quilting. Her son was a few months older than H and I was pregnant with Pops, so we'd supped plenty of tea and coffee at a number of coffee mornings for the dispossessed – I mean new mums.

We had also become founder members of a patchwork group called The Evening Stars – yes, because we came out at night! - where we met a bunch of women who also loved cutting up large bits of fabric, into small bits, and sewing them back together again. We were a diverse bunch of mixed ages, backgrounds and experiences yet I had never found quite so much acceptance as within The Evening Stars.

Much like I imagine women gathered in times past – though we've moved on from candles – we sat and sewed and talked. Wonderful patchwork quilts were created and discussed, skills shared, laughter laughed and, *Little House on The Prairie* moments aside, it was a great bunch of women, many of whom still sew together.

Chris and I had had to take it a stage further. We became fabriholics, frequenting any cloth sale within a 'reasonable' distance, amassing piles of one hundred per cent cotton like misers hoard gold. H and Pops had experienced a childhood trailing around fabric sales, patchwork shops and quilting exhibitions wherever we went. It was a life saver, it gave us some structure and helped keep me sane through several shattering years. The Evening Stars remain a bunch of strong, supportive wise women who know how to use a needle to best effect.

I don't know what was in Chris's head as she surveyed the room, took in the state of both my children, the seriousness of the situation. But doers *'do'* and it wasn't long before we were over the emotional bit – sort of – and on to the practical side.

'You need a new phone,' said Chris, 'have you thought about a contract?'

My face answered the question.

'OK. I can pop into town and get you a new pay-as-you-go,' said Chris. 'Yes, it will be the simplest, cheapest one I can find!'

'Right, what else do you need?' And she was off.

It wasn't long before Pops had her own bottle of Calpol, and I had Paracetamol, Tampons and hand wash for clothes. We also established all H wanted was linguine with fresh tomato sauce and peas. Neither of us knew Bristol, so had no idea where to head for *'Pasta Central'*. Chris called her Techy Husband, who soon had a location and directions to the nearest Italian.

H only managed a forkful but the whole adventure was such an 'everything is possible' moment, it gave us an enormous boost.

By the time Chris had returned with a foil tray full of pasta it was dark. Doctor John told me the hospital had booked a room in a nearby hotel, regularly used by the hospital authorities, so Pops had somewhere to stay that night. I resisted the urge to say 'what, on her own?' It was implicit I would be staying with her. I still could not get my head around the concept I was expected to leave my son, in this state, on his own, overnight. It went against every single one of my mothering instincts.

If Chris had not been there, I don't know what I would have done. I could no more have left H alone than danced *Swan Lake* in a size ten tutu. I was given a computer printout with a reference number on it, the name of a hotel with an 'it's over there' (thank goodness for Techy Husband on the end of the phone) and told it was paid for by the hospital account. All we had to do was check in.

I had no choice. Pops would have to go with Chris and they would both stay in the hotel overnight. My mothering instincts - the ones screaming *but Pops is poorly and wants her mummy* – had to be tossed out the window.

My seven-year-old, swine flu-ridden daughter had to be bundled up like something someone had left on a train, end up in *Hotel of the Homeless and Stateless, on Somewhere Street, Nowhere Corner.* I was distraught. I think it was only because Pops was so poorly – that's right, send her out in the cold and dark away from her mum – she took Chris's hand without a whimper. All she had with her were Leemy (her stuffed monkey), pyjamas, a toothbrush, clean knickers and a bottle of Calpol. There was no point sending her off with a hairbrush, she wouldn't let Chris brush her hair anyway. It had only been cut once since she was born. It was one of our bedtime rituals, brushing out the plait she could sit on.

Oh please let my phone hold out so I can speak to Pops, I begged a silent entity. *Let me be able to say goodnight to my daughter. Please!*

'It's good *Auntie Chris* is here,' said H. How did my nine-year old know exactly the right thing to say? We had never called Chris *'Auntie Chris'.* She has been *Auntie Chris* ever since that day.

When I spoke to Pops, after they arrived at the hotel, she was tearful. Surely it couldn't be right to send a seven-year-old, with swine flu, into a busy hotel?

Meanwhile, in Room 4, H's oxygen levels were stable, but not high enough. His breathing seemed laboured and his face looked even more gaunt, accentuated as it was by his glasses, which seemed to have grown in proportion to his shrinking face.

Would the phone ever stop ringing? Another request to visit. But I couldn't let people see H like this. I knew I could not cope with their reactions, particularly my mother, seeing her only grandson, her first grandchild, looking like this. It was hard enough for me to see and I'd been in on it since the beginning. I knew I did not have the strength to reassure other people all would be well. Was it fair to liken his appearance to that of a Belsen survivor? Fair or not, that's what he looked like.

At no point did it occur to me my family wanted to see H before he died.

CHAPTER FOURTEEN

OUR VIEW ON THE WORLD WAS REDUCED TO A SMALL, NARROW, METAL latticed window of *safety glass* in the door, a metal framed window, with a knackered latch, which looked out on to the main road. It was suffocating.

I could see - and hear – the main road. I could see buildings, funky shop fronts, church spires on the horizon. I stared out of the window. Was this what it was like to be locked in a city prison cell?

I had often wondered how that must feel, to be imprisoned, to look out on a scurrying world. You don't 'scurry' on the inside. So often in Reading I had driven past the former incarnation of the town's 'gaol', once home to Oscar Wilde and Hollywood star Stacy Keach, and wondered what it must feel like, to be locked up, contained within brick. Now, I knew. Except we had no parole date, no solicitor; you only get those when you commit a crime.

I looked out of the window. The sky, grey of course, had definitely shrunk.

Do you ever look up at the sky? Have you noticed how, in built up places, when you are surrounded by the lines of living and working, hemmed in by the very fabric which shapes big towns and huge cities, you don't see much sky? You can look up, of course you can look up. The shape of a roof, the line of bricks defining a Victorian apex, an architect designed sheet of glass and metal, a contour created by the coming together of two office blocks and an express supermarket – they steal the sky.

Everything was gone from our lives. Everything had been removed. All we had left was what we had now, at that very moment, in Room 4. I felt I'd even lost the sky. Our huge, never-ending, limitless skies over Dartmoor, those which gently lapped the edges of the sea as far as the eye could see; the blue expanses which framed sandy beaches and made rocks shine like salty diamonds. It all was gone.

Then I remembered. Pops' middle name, 'Sky'. Without the 'e'; plain Sky. How could I think in terms of losing the sky, my Pops Sky? If I didn't find a way of keeping her in Bristol, finding a way of caring for her in Bristol, she would be removed too.

I will not lose anything more! Screamed the angry voice in my head. I need to be the mother my children need. I can't whine about grey skies.

That night, lying on the pull-down bed, I didn't sleep. My past played out. As if I was a drowning woman?

From childhood, failed relationships, travel, people, childbirth, divorce, houses, quilts even memorable meals. My mind had gone into *filing cabinet* mode. Counting sheep is dull, much better to count life events, try and cheer yourself up, fathom why your life has crashed into a brick wall, then fallen down a black hole.

Forget the failures, said head. Learn from them. Allow the good bits to power up the future. Someone out there must be able to help.

H was awake. I helped him use a pee bottle, left it by the door. A nurse came. She went. Another came, took H's temperature, checked his oxygen levels.

'I'm going to call a doctor,' she said.

By the early hours of the morning, I'd lost count of how many doctors had been through Room 4. I wished I'd had proper pyjamas. A strappy tee shirt and a long black crocheted cardigan were highly unsuitable night attire for a public hospital room. I didn't own any pyjamas. Having three doctors in the room at once, talking in low voices, put pyjamas out of my mind.

By morning I felt like the walking dead. H looked it. Well, he was lying down, but air of *zombie* hung heavy. But I'd had my Eureka! moment. Cousin Debbie! Of all the people I'd ever known she was the one. The one person who might, just might, be able to help.

My mum and ex-mum-in-law were already carers, of sick spouses. My brother had a full-time job running his own company. Their dad worked full-time and was somewhat challenged in the parenting department anyway, on the grounds of no experience.

My friends are my friends because they lead busy, fulfilling lives, which meant they were all bringing up their own children or had chosen not to reproduce because they wanted to nurture careers instead. No one could just drop out of their life, to come and look after Pops. Except, possibly, Cousin Debbie. Being my eldest cousin, her children were at university and she ran her own, highly successful soft furnishings business. I knew she was busy, but maybe she would be able to help.

I rang my mum and asked her to ring Cousin Debbie.

'Ask her mum, ask her, please. She's the only person I can think of. Even if it's just for a few days it will give me a chance to think of something. There is no one else.'

In desperation I'd even rung a Devon friend who worked as a professional carer, asked her if she would consider working in Bristol, I'd raise the money to pay her. But of course she couldn't, her sons were the same ages as my two – how could she leave them with her husband? Most mums can't walk away from young families. I knew that, but I was desperate.

The smell of hospital was beginning to get to me. I think the more tired I became the harder the airlessness was to cope with. I opened the window, rush hour roared in. A quick reminder the sky still existed and I was back with stale breath, farting cabbages, eau de vomit and the distinct aroma of disinfectant battling with mass produced food. Pass the essential oils!

Just as I began to fixate on the *click click click* of the oxygen machine, Pops and Chris walked in through the door. I could breathe again. My daughter was back.

It was Friday. The docs were going to start H on chemo. Chris disappeared into Bristol, to get me a new phone. Pops was sprawled on the pull-down bed.

It was time. Time to shut up and buckle up. Today H would start his first round of chemotherapy, described by doctors as a *roller coaster*. I'm terrified of roller coasters, even tiny ones. Here goes...

Well, first a bit of waiting. More waiting. Bit more. A morning's worth as it turned out.

'Could I sign the consent form please?' said someone, the form signed by a doctor called Cummins, of whom I still have absolutely no recollection.

Under serious or frequently occurring risks he/she listed: infections, mucositis, cardiotoxicity, liver dysfunction, fevers, rashes, nausea and vomiting, hair loss, second malignancy.

In this pink form – *to be completed using black/blue ballpoint pen press hard to ensure a legible copy* – I was being asked to allow doctors to make my son very ill indeed. There is a reason why chemotherapy is called *the killing cure*. But what are you going to say at that point? *'No thanks, I'll give him a couple of Aspirin'.*

Yet again I had no choice and yet again I had to agree to something which went against every single one of my mothering instincts.

It was November 2009, a week after my son's ninth birthday, and I'd just signed a form allowing doctors to pump him full of drugs which could kill him. At the very least he would lose all his hair.

If I didn't agree, he would die anyway.

CHAPTER FIFTEEN

MY NEW BEST FRIENDS HAD BECOME *CYTOSINE ARABINOSIDE*, *Daunombicin* and *Etoposide* – ADE for short. The first round of chemotherapy was designed to induce remission from the leukaemia, which meant killing off everything in H's blood, including the good stuff, like all his immunity.

A blue, high sided plastic tray was carried in by a nurse who wore, in addition to the anti-swine flu get up, a pair of plastic disposable protective cuffs up to her elbow and an enormous pair of protective plastic glasses, covering half her face.

The drugs themselves were highly toxic on the skin and I was warned from the arrival of that first tray I had to wear latex gloves each time I cleared up any of my son's bodily fluids.

I tried to count the number of syringes in the blue tray, but there were too many. I don't think H was really taking notice of anything much by that stage. One drip stand was not enough, so another was found. At what point would the medics find another body, because this one couldn't cope? Well, that was pretty crap black humour, said voice in head.

It didn't take long for things to start happening.

'We can give him drugs for the sickness,' said a nurse.

Shame they couldn't for the diarrhoea.

Cardboard containers – filled with sick, wee and pooh - began to stack up by the door out of Room 4, alongside uneaten trays of food and a pile of soiled laundry. My favourite scarf - which had so often been used as a blanket or sun protector for both my children – fell off a hook and into a bowl of toxic pooh. Should I wash it, or bin it? What would you have done?

There was too much sentiment attached to that scarf, it had to be saved. In washing it, while wearing latex gloves, I discovered the shower room toilet made a good drying room. Knickers joined scarf.

H had no clean pyjamas left, but there would have been no point him wearing any. It was impossible to miss how powerful the drugs were. I kept telling myself over and over it was what the chemotherapy was supposed to do.

A tall man came into the room. 'Hello,' said a friendly Scottish accent 'I'm Jamie.'

Jamie wasn't a myth! He really existed!

So many people had mentioned Jamie but by then, I'd assumed we weren't on his agenda. Now here he was, his handshake too warm to belong to a hologram, the crinkle of the plastic apron and his masked face a reality we couldn't escape.

Someone, somewhere, must have briefed Jamie. He told me he was the Leukaemia Nurse Specialist, and he was there to answer any questions I might have - and to see what could be done to help us.

I'm sure Jamie did get a word in edgeways. By the time he left we had certainly leapt off the page of whichever file he'd been looking through. He got the extended litany about no help available in the family, ex-husband's court order, even though I felt like a broken record which increasingly just made me feel like my life was just one big piece of crap.

Jamie said he was there to help us through. Jamie felt like James Bond. He said he knew how hard this must be, alluding to his own childhood. It was not hard to have faith in this charming, straight-talking, father of two.

Jamie said the hotel issue would be sorted and for the next few nights the hospital would pay the bill, until something else could be sorted, now CLIC House was no longer an option because of the swine flu.

'All we need is a small mattress for Pops,' I said. 'I've worked it all out. There's space in the shower room for her.'

H was the priority, said Jamie. He would be very closely monitored, particularly as the swine flu had complicated things. He underlined the doctors in Bristol had a wealth of knowledge, were highly experienced in the use of antibiotics and antifungals.

Jamie also emphasised Ward 34 was a 24/7 entity. I knew that already; each minute was a day, each day an hour, seconds had become invisible markers whether it was day, night or something in between. Time no longer had any of the familiar markers found on any clock. It was one continuous piece of nothing with no beginning and no end. Just one long *wait...* Punctuated with a string of crisis of varying severity. No thrill of a Tardis.

Yet I felt Jamie was suggesting our situation did have options. His leukaemia knowledge was clearly enormous, his confidence was laced with words like 'possible', 'doable' and 'way forward'.

As soon as he arrived, Jamie seemed to be gone, leaving behind the 'smell' of calm – or was it fabric softener mixed with aftershave? - much like a glamorous woman leaves behind the whiff of an expensive perfume.

Jamie's visit didn't stop the effluent piling up by the door. I began to feel increasingly helpless, despite meeting Jamie. I couldn't take anything to the sluice room, because of my swine flu. All the cardboard containers had to go there, each one marked in permanent black marker with H's name, pooh, wee and sick weighed so doctors could measure input against output. I became very anxious about the increasing pile of waste and decaying food. Had the meaning of the word *sterile* changed since we'd arrived in Bristol?

In reality it meant Ward 34 was a very busy ward. I had no measure of it, no idea staffing levels were sometimes unable to deal with the amount of work sick children entail. Was every room on Ward 34 like this? Nurses were sometimes chatty, other times in and out faster than the cats after a flea treatment.

My agitation at H not eating and barely drinking, took over. Keeping him hydrated became my focus, which was tough with no direct access to water, shop or fridge.

Pops was sleepy. H was out of it. Chris came back with a new mobile for me. Figuring out how it worked took up time, especially as it didn't seem to stop ringing.

A woman wearing an ethnic style cardigan, which could have been hand knitted, came into the room, cautiously.

'Hello, you must be Sharon. I'm Lin, your CLIC social worker.' I could see her eyes; they were flecked with wisdom.

I invited Lin into my 'office', the toilet with the seat down. We could only laugh about it. Good start, I figured; sense of humour.

Poor Lin, she got the brunt of my confusion. Somehow, she seemed to be making sense of my outpourings. I was trying to summarise, give her as much info as I could, journalist persona in overdrive.

Lin gave me a CLIC Sargent Filofax, leaflets and some reassurance she would investigate what options were open to me, her words 'temporary foster care' penetrated my monologue.

'Pops is not going into foster care. Why would I want complete strangers caring for my daughter? All I need is a small child's mattress. I've worked it all out. She can even use this bathroom as a separate bedroom, there is room with a small mattress.'

Little could be achieved late on a Friday afternoon, but Lin said she could apply for a £180-pound grant from a cancer charity for us, was it OK for her to do that? I said, *'yes please'.* It would really help.

Lin said she would see me next week. She told me she worked part time but added there was a CLIC team based in the hospital.

'Arthur?' said Lin. 'No, I'm not sure I know an Arthur. I work for the CLIC Sargent team of social workers. He may be attached to the hospital. I don't know him. I'll see you next week.'

I liked Lin; felt she had listened to me. I was very grateful she hadn't left with a cheery *'have a good weekend'.*

The day limped towards evening and Pops said she didn't want to go to the hotel with Chris, she wanted to stay with me. I knew how she felt, the swine flu was taking its toll.

A new nurse arrived on the scene, said Pops should be going. I wasn't sure at first if she was being compassionate towards Pops, or simply trying to get her out of the room. It didn't take long to work out she wanted Pops out. Pops didn't want to leave. I didn't want her to go – she needed me. I needed to know she was OK.

New nurse was a Nasty Nurse.

'You have to take your daughter to the hotel. It's all paid for. It's time to go,' she said.

'But she doesn't want to go,' I said, 'she's got swine flu.'

Another game of verbal ping-pong was underway. The 'You have to go to CLIC House' scenario; round two.

I rang my Reading friend, Dr Leather. She's a psychologist and not for the first time my *voice of reason.*

'Cathy, what do I do? This is so hard. Pops doesn't want to go. I don't want her to go. She's really poorly and she just wants to be with me. Why can't the hospital see that?'

'You have to cooperate with them,' said Cathy. 'You have to be seen to be trying to find solutions and they have made provision for you. If you cooperate now it will be much easier for you to negotiate in the future. You must cooperate, that way they will be more amenable to helping you.'

I knew Cathy was right, but it didn't make it any easier. I couldn't leave H. He was far too ill. Pops was also ill - and distraught.

Nasty Nurse came back to Room 4. 'Your daughter needs to go,' she said, 'she can't stay here'.

'Can't you see she's ill?' I said. 'She doesn't want to leave me, I'm her mum. Have you no humanity?' My voice was cracking, tears close by. But I did manage to make my feelings very clear.

Nasty Nurse turned on her heel – yes, just like all the best villains she made a proper exit - with a final flourish of 'Well she can't stay here.'

By then I was feeling sorry for Chris, too. Sat in the room she was now a part of the drama.

'If we go now,' said Chris, 'we can call you from the hotel room. Maybe it will give Pops a chance to get a good night's sleep. And the room's all sorted and paid for. We'll be back first thing.'

I put Pops in her coat, gave her a big cuddle and told her I'd speak to her on Auntie Chris's phone as soon as she was in her pyjamas.

I thought it was only men who were supposed to break your heart in two, smash up the pieces and then scatter them around the shared memory garden of your soul.

My heart had just been ripped out by some faceless dimwits and it was now somewhere else, beating, keeping me going remotely. My sick seven-year-old daughter had been sent out into a cold dark night, for a second time, to stay in a strange hotel room with someone who wasn't her mum. I felt hollow. Actually, truly empty inside.

I had to turn my mind to her brother, who was being sick again.

It wasn't long before I got a phone call. I even managed to find the right button to press so I could answer it.

'Sorry to call Sharon,' said Chris, 'but the hotel receptionist is denying all knowledge of a booking from the hospital. I've given them the reference number and said we stayed last night, gave them the room number and everything. She's adamant we can't stay unless I pay for a room.'

CHAPTER SIXTEEN

I experienced a moment of utter fury. The image of Pops stood by the hotel reception desk, holding Leemy, and huddled in her coat just wanting me to tuck her into bed, took over.

'Can you cover it Chris, and I'll sort it this end. I'll pay for the room, one way or another.'

I knew Chris didn't have much money; Techy Husband had just been made redundant. How could the hospital authorities be so cruel, so bloody useless?

Reality check – the hospital is here to heal H, not deal with domestic difficulties, said inner voice. Somehow, appreciating that didn't make any of this easier, particularly as I felt they were the ones who had actively created this particular domestic difficulty.

I wanted to go and get Pops, bring her back here, bed her down and give Nasty Nurse – who appeared to have gone off duty, never to be seen again – a verbal two fingers she'd never forget.

If I'd been a convicted criminal, people would have shown more humanity towards us. (or so I thought, back then ...) I'd been in prison, for six weeks, spent my 21st inside – as a student observer, in case you're wondering – so I knew murderers, drug dealers and thieves were being treated more humanely than we were. (There's the middle-class ignorance kicking in!) At least in prison you get a gym and a library. What did we have? Enforced separation, incarceration, a sink, a toilet and a shower, no access to drinking water and months of fear and suffering lined up. And all obtained with no criminal record. Well, not yet ...

I'd never been in such a tight spot as this, but I had lived enough to appreciate getting angry was not going to help. I'd have to gather my thoughts as a General would gather his army, form a strategy, read up on my subject and stay strong. Whatever that meant. I didn't feel 'strong'. I'm convinced 'being strong' weakens you, over time. But if 'being strong' meant keeping going, staying calm and fighting for both my children, then I'd be 'strong'.

I sat on the edge of the fold down bed, not relishing the thought of another sweaty night stuck to a plastic mattress.

Stop being so ungrateful and get on with it, said voice in head. If we were truly refugees none of us would have had a bed that night. None of us were really eating anything but there was, somehow, food out there. We still had a home (abandoned), a life (abandoned), people who loved us. We lived in one of the freest societies in the world and, most importantly, H was plugged into a highly experienced medical team who were going to save his life. We'd just lost our feature slot on page five of the Refugee Times.

Funny how we often have everything we need, yet feel we have nothing. I don't mean 'I've got nothing to wear'. Or 'there's nothing in the fridge'. I mean we, all of us, too often spend time focusing on what we 'don't' have rather than what we 'do' have.

I had never had a lot, but always had enough, plus a bit. Brought up by two parents who had lived through World War Two meant life was never extravagant; but there was always enough. And holidays! We didn't always get what we wanted or wanted what we got. But it was the way things were and I think most of my peers were also content with their lot. I grew up in an affluent town, had a solid education and virtually all of us went on to university and built careers. I had plenty.

Fair to say though, my upbringing was, in a word, *ordinary.*

By my twenties, the eighties and Thatcher's Britain were in full flow. Consumerism and shoulder pads were hot news before the softer, greener nineties hit. I worked hard, played hard, used my passport whenever possible.

Being a cub reporter on a local paper paid shared bills and funded weekends, with the help of an overdraft. As my unremarkable rise through the ranks took me into the world of court reporting, a fascinating world where humanity is offered up on a plate – a very large plate – I found myself on a collision course with a ticking biological clock. Marriage, birth, divorce and a whole new incarnation followed.

Sitting on a plastic mattress in Bristol Children's Hospital, nursing a very sick boy surgically attached to so many plastic tubes they were impossible to keep track of - while frantic about my other child, sick in an unknown hotel room in a strange city - had never been part of my life plan. Though granted, 'plan' was a bit of an exaggeration.

Moving from Berkshire to Devon had been a major life choice two years in the making, my mind made up after I drove H and Pops – then five and six years old – out to the stunning Italian mountains of Les Marches, for a family party.

If I could do that, I told myself, moving almost 200 miles up the road was possible.

People back then had called me *mad.* When they saw how settled, how content – how *at home* - we were in the West Country, they told me I was *strong.*

Back then I had a choice. My son getting cancer at the age of nine, was not a choice.

I had convinced myself before driving to Italy, that if I was capable of driving a borrowed seven-and-a-half-ton truck out to the Ukraine– the only time I'll probably ever drive a Mercedes – I could certainly 'do' Europe in a car, with my children. Top tip: it stops the 'Are we nearly there yet' syndrome, when you can respond with a swift, 'It's not as far as Italy!'

I had to believe if I could move my small and imperfectly formed family from the Home Counties, leave behind all our support networks, start a new life in Devon, then six months living by a hospital bedside, in a strange city, was possible.

It felt like we had nothing. Yet we were in a situation where we had everything we needed – to get H well.

The phone rang. 'It's OK, it's OK Sharon. She's a bit upset but we've had a chat and Pops' going to get into bed in a minute,' said my stoic friend Chris. It wasn't hard to pick up on her angst.

'Mummy, it's Pops. I want to come back to the hospital; please can I sleep with you mummy? I'll curl up really small, you won't know I'm there,' sobbed Pops.

'Oh Luvvy, we're not allowed to do that. Anyway, I bet the hotel's exciting,' I said, yet again horrified at the words coming out of my mouth.

'I just want to come back to the hospital. Please mummy!' said Pops.

If H hadn't been throwing up at that moment, I would have gone and got my daughter. I did my best to reassure her. Chris texted me soon after to say she was asleep.

But I couldn't go and get my daughter. I didn't know where she was.

CHAPTER
SEVENTEEN

SOMETHING DIED INSIDE ME THAT NIGHT. SOME SMALL AND HIDDEN PART of me, the part which had always believed *things would turn out OK because it wasn't really that bad.*

I was alone. I thought I'd known that. In all the times I'd felt lonely, or struggled, or been scared that I was responsible for bringing up two children on my own - I'd always believed *things would turn out OK.* I had always felt there was a way. A future. A solution. I'd just got on with it.

When it looked like we three would lose our home to an embittered ex-husband, the home I'd worked so hard for; when I lost a baby and thought I'd never be able to have another one; when my grandma died; the first time my heart broke; the job I wanted so desperately but didn't get. Each time I'd had the belief *everything would be OK.* And besides, disappointment is part of life, said my mum, because *life's not fair.*

Every time I'd found a way through. And each time I'd soldered a bit of wisdom on to the suit of armour I had learnt to wear as a child, the one which protected my soft, Piscean, inner core. The tough outer coating was always padded out with a lust for travel, adventure and people who shared my taste in chain mail. And it was all held together by the belief that *things would turn out OK.*

That Friday night into day, that blurring of one set of events straight into another, stole a part of me away. It was like a physical pain I couldn't touch.

H had been almost eighteen months old when Pops was born, a second emergency Caesarean. Caring for them both, day after day changing two sets of nappies, on crutches at one point, because my back gave up, feeding two utterly dependent beings, attending birthday parties, throwing birthday parties, functioning socially as a threesome, barely ever functioning socially as an adult.

During those years I met an awful lot of women, some are still friends. Pasta became as essential as the washing machine. I grew alongside my children and we had adventures even when there were days when the furthest I was able to manage was the paper shop on the corner, pushing the double buggy; to buy a newspaper I never got the chance to read. Sometimes those were the good days.

The pressures of an aggressive divorce solicitor, the fear of homelessness, a fractured relationship with my family, no money. They all made life harder. But I had always believed *things would be OK.* And I'd always found a way.

Then we moved to Devon and life had begun to find some balance again. We had begun to stabilise, walk the tightrope with a little confidence. See the horizon, breath in the sky, believe in a future. Hell, have time to think there was a future instead of just one day after another.

However hard those early days were, blurred by exhaustion, I always knew I had chosen to be a mother. It was me who divorced my now ex-husband, because I knew I could not make our marriage work and it would have become more and more painful, more destructive for both of us.

I loved loving my children. I had incredible support from a handful of people who really cared. I was also resourceful, could budget my way out of a crisis - thanks to the excellent training from my mum - and count laughing as one of my favourite hobbies. Sewing was sanity.

All of this meant H, Pops and I were an incredibly close, tight-knit family who trusted each other implicitly.

On the day my son started chemotherapy, something inside me died. I didn't know *everything would be OK,* ever again

My seven-year-old daughter had been taken away from me and my nine-year old son had cancer. I felt our tightrope had snapped.

CHAPTER
EIGHTEEN

Lying on the pull-down bed, staring up at the ceiling, I could see the bright, dark blue light of a new day throwing the hanging strips of the blind, dangling across the window, into sharper focus.

I'd had to open the window; H's temperature had rocketed again in the night. Where were all the cars going to so early on a Saturday morning?

An electric fan was now competing for attention with the *click click click* of the oxygen machine, along with the *tic tic tic* of an electric syringe driver pumping H full of pain relief, or chemo or anti something-or-other.

An alarm went off on one of the pumps attached to my son. They were programmed to go off when a medication was finished, or when the tube had blocked. I had already learnt to fear the alarms, terrified an air bubble would worm its way into a tube and get in to his system. It was irrational, but so was our entire situation. My psyche was on permanent overdrive. Lack of food and sleep wasn't helping, but I couldn't eat, and sleep had been replaced by short periods of unconsciousness.

The new day was grey. The Tamiflu was making it feel as if

someone had turned my nostrils inside out and dried them out on a rack in the oven, gas mark low, overnight.

It hadn't made me feel any less flu-like but at least I had avoided any nausea, vomiting, skin rashes, hives, blisters, itching and swelling of the face, eyes, lips tongue or throat. It really wouldn't have been fair to compete with H. Pops had avoided abnormal behaviours (including shaking, confusion, speech problems, seizures, hearing voices or hallucinations) that could lead to death, because I'd refused to let her take the Tamiflu. No wonder the doctors hadn't tried to persuade me otherwise.

I just wanted to see Pops, give her a hug. I knew Chris was bringing her early because, between making quilts and hoarding fabric, she was a playwright and was currently directing a show. The plan was for her to drive back to Reading, attend various meetings and then drive back to Bristol to look after Pops that night. I could only think, '*above and beyond*'. I was still waiting on a phone call from mum, to hear if she had been able to speak to Cousin Debbie. I couldn't think beyond tonight. It meant I only had to worry about the next hour.

When Pops arrived, she looked as if she was carrying the weight of a thousand toy boxes on her shoulders. Her eyes were all puffy and shrouded in dark circles. I took off her coat, wrapped her in a blanket and sat her on my lap. I'm not really sure who was hanging on to who.

Chris disappeared. A stream of people came and went. I put Pops in the pull-down bed. A tray of food appeared. I put it by the door, alongside the other effluent. Another high sided blue tray arrived, carried by a nurse wearing white plastic arm cuffs. And a mask.

Someone told me the hotel had been sorted out, they would reimburse Chris.

When H declared an interest in eating some kiwi fruit, I was elated! I think it was discovering that our *Devon Fridge Supplies,* handily secreted in a shoulder bag almost a week ago, had finally perished, which probably tipped me over the edge.

One of our loveliest nurses came into the room. I still didn't really know what Rachel looked like, as half her face was covered in a paper mask. But it wasn't hard to tell I freaked her out.

'Rachel, if I keep pressing the help button over there,' I said, 'pointing to the square red button on the electrical over bed headboard, 'does it jeopardise care for any other child?'

Clearly puzzled she said it didn't.

'So, what does it do? Does it get people into the room?' I said.

'Well, yes – if you need help someone will come,' she said.

'Right,' I said. 'I'm going to start pressing that button and I'm not going to stop pressing it until someone comes to talk to me. I want to talk to someone who can help us.

'No one is realising what our situation is. No one gets it. We're trapped in this hospital room and no one is listening. I'm sure the friends I still have on newspapers in London would be very interested to hear about what's going on in Bristol Children's Hospital! You won't know this but I was a journalist. This would make good headlines,' I said, knowing it to be true.

Clearly shocked, Rachel's eyes widened.

'I do hear what you're saying, Sharon. But pressing the buzzer won't help. It just goes to the nurses' station. And there's only two of us on duty.'

I ended up pressing the buzzer an awful lot that afternoon. Not because I was being a right cow, but because H was deteriorating. There was no way the nurses on duty could forget we were there.

I pressed it when we needed clean sheets. When we ran out of cardboard wee bottles. When the pile of effluent built up, for more drinking water, for cleaning wipes, disposable bottom pads. By then the diarrhoea was simply pouring out of H's bum, which was getting redder and redder.

I pressed the buzzer.

'Can I have some cream for his bottom?'

Could we have some DVDs please? I pressed the buzzer.

We'd run out of plastic cups and each time I tried to give H water the cup had to be thrown away. I pressed the buzzer.

What time was the next medication due?

I pressed the buzzer.

Why hadn't the next bit of chemo arrived?

I pressed the buzzer.

The alarm on the pump was going off.

I pressed the buzzer.

H's temperature had shot up again. I pressed the buzzer.

The alarm; the buzzer.

Each press of the buzzer became a scream, inside my head. An attempt to reach out in the hope someone, somewhere, would see what was happening.

Yet each press of the buzzer was also a need and it made me understand how helpless we were. There was not a single thing I could do for my children except be there; be mum. I was so thirsty. No one brought water. The nurses were simply too busy. H needed water. I knew I was dehydrating. I gave Pops a carton of hospital orange juice; sweet, cheap, syrupy, the kind of tooth rot I would never buy.

What was I supposed to do? How was I supposed to cope with this crisis? What madness written in to the hospital rules stated mothers and children are allowed to be ripped apart at a time of such acute need? Especially when there is a solution to hand. In the form of a small mattress.

How had all those mothers, forced into Victorian workhouses, coped? There is a reason why poverty, crime and prostitution go hand in hand. Would hospital isolation be a defence in court today?

If I'd been in a locked cell, I would have started slamming the small door shutter up and down, up and down, up and down. Until someone came. Until someone DID something. Until a solicitor was called. Until proper contact with the outside world was established.

I'd make a very bad prisoner. I was being a bad hospital inmate and I wasn't even a patient.

In here, in Room 4, Ward 34, somewhere in Bristol, we were invisible. How could I make anyone listen?

There was not a single person out there who could arrive, at the prison gates – I mean hospital doors – unannounced and stick up for us. Shout for us. Tell the management team it was an unacceptable way to treat a traumatised family. It even occurred to me I should contact Amnesty International. Except we weren't international. We had no rights. We had done nothing wrong either. But this was happening in England in the middle of a large city full of charities helping people. A cultured city full of art and music and middle-class people.

I wasn't angry at the cancer. There was no point in being angry with a disease. You have to confront it. Stare it in the face and get on with it. And we were. H was being incredible.

I was angry with the faceless ones, the policy makers who were refusing to see what was happening, pretending our situation was acceptable, burying the truth of it. I couldn't help feeling I'd been too bloody polite.

I pressed the buzzer, motivated by all our thirsts.

What if I got some handcuffs, locked Pops and me together and then locked us to H's bed? Now that would make headlines. Then we couldn't be ignored. If I didn't draw attention to our situation, no one else would.

I was becoming increasingly desperate. Feeling insignificant is not an issue for me. I've had years of practice; but being insignificant when you need help, when you need support, when your situation is so desperate even with a degree in 'Getting out of

Tight Spots', and a PhD in 'Thinking Outside the Box', you can't find a solution – being insignificant is not helpful.

When it seemed things really couldn't get any worse, Rachel came back. She sat down on the spare chair.

'I've spoken to someone,' said Rachel, 'a consultant I know, called Helen. She's really lovely, Sharon, she'll be able to listen. But she's not on duty until tomorrow. She may be able to help.'

I thanked Rachel and apologised for the buzzer stunt comment. 'I'm getting desperate Rachel; I don't know what to do. I don't want to be a newspaper headline. They want to take Pops into foster care,' and I burbled my way to tears. 'I won't let that happen. I won't!'

Forget *road rage* – could that have been the first ever *room rage? Womb rage* even? 'Back away from my children', screeched voice in head. If I'd been a lioness I would have attacked by now. Instead, all I'd been able to do was threaten to press a small red button, and keep pressing and pressing, until someone came.

I already knew the world didn't contain big red alarm buttons, bells alerting help squads. If it did, I'd have pressed one long before we'd arrived in Bristol.

Rachel came back with my very own box of hospital issue tissues, white. It was the loveliest thing anyone could possibly have done at that moment in time.

CHAPTER NINETEEN

I HAD SO OFTEN FELT, SINCE CHILDHOOD, I WAS LOOKING ON, FROM THE outside. Yet now I'm on the inside, looking out. I prefer the view I am used to.

Here I'm not me. I'm 'mum', a nameless patient's mother, a faceless person with little more than a three pack of M&S knickers, an electric toothbrush I couldn't charge and months of uncertainty stretching ahead.

You want to know what fear is? Fear is the thought of losing your son and daughter – one to cancer, the other to bureaucracy. Fear is losing control of every element of your life, not knowing when you will ever see your home again, or if the life you have worked so hard for can possibly survive. Fear is a stranger's sneeze in a lift.

We humans are designed to fight fear. It is built in as the 'fight or flight' mechanism and these chemicals, pumping around our strong frail bodies, work. Now I feared how long I could keep going. The fight had mullered the flight alright, but would the fight coursing through my veins overwhelm the last vestiges of my sanity? How do you *'stay strong'*?

A friend had asked me that day how I was keeping going. My response was instinctive.

'I'm fighting for my children. I'm the only one who can.'

I was a faceless, nameless mum and so were all the others on the ward. We parents all kept going because we had no choice. I was no different. We were all getting through each day, however we could. Even though I didn't know any of the other parents, I knew it must have been the same for them.

If I left Bristol a size twelve with obsessive compulsive cleaning habits, I'd embrace that – fat chance.

All I really wanted was to take both my children home and get on with our small and humble lives in our small and humble Devon town. My sofa. I wanted my sofa and my open fire. I wanted to light candles and watch rubbish TV.

Instead, I was perched like a pixie, legs under chin, on the edge of a plastic mattress in a small, cold, noisy hospital room looking over at my son who was sleeping fitfully between hospital white sheets. I wanted my daughter. I wanted to cuddle away her tears. Mine streamed, relentless, onto an institutional floor I could only pray was clean. The world into which the three of us had been plunged was a secret, hidden, unknown world. The world of childhood cancer.

We were one of just ten daily diagnoses. One family out of a statistical handful.

It meant I was even more on the outside looking in. When this was over – whichever way it went – we would be different. We would be even more on the outside. It would become even harder to look in and see myself alongside everyone else.

What's that famous quote? The future is a strange land? All three of our futures were beginning to look like alien landscapes. If I couldn't find a practical solution for Pops the hospital bureaucrats were forming opinions of their own. If I couldn't find a night time carer for Pops, they were looking at a radical solution.

Pops, my seven-year-old daughter who had done nothing wrong and was loved and cared for and nurtured by me, and her brother – would have to go into temporary foster care. The very thought if it became a physical pain. I simply could not let that happen. I would not allow my daughter to be handed over to the care of complete strangers. OVER MY DEAD BODY.

I was being forced to deal not just with my nine-year old son's cancer, which could kill him. But I was being forced to make a choice between my children. If I stayed with H at night – and there was no way I could leave him when he was suffering so much – then I could not care for my daughter. And Pops needed me more than ever. This could not be right.

Our lives had become a series of film titles. We had gone from 'The Perfect Storm' (with no George Clooney in sight) to 'Sophie's Choice' (I had to become tougher than Meryl Streep in all her film roles combined). And these were not my analogies. They were observations from hospital staff.

Between stifled sobs I recapped. We'd gone from swine flu to leukaemia. Were now imprisoned in a hospital room on the fifth floor – yes, fifth floor, I now knew which floor we were on, I asked a nurse - of a large hospital in a city we'd never been to, surrounded by masked men and women. My son could die and now the bureaucrats wanted to take my daughter away, hand her over to strangers. A mythical social worker called 'Arthur' had still made no contact. Our home, car and two cats were almost 90 miles up the road and I felt I was in imminent danger of losing my marbles.

The realisation I was rocking backwards and forwards, tears streaming down my face, fist in mouth so I couldn't scream – I'm not painting an image, that's how I found myself when the remaining brain cells kicked in – brought me to my senses.

There was a way through all this. There had to be. I just had to find it.

It was 4.30am. H was asleep and I was hanging on to the plot much like an international super hero would be holding on to the plane controls to avoid it crashing into a small village. No crashes for me. Hold on girl, you're not in the straight jacket quite yet. BOTH my children needed me. I would find a way to be there for BOTH of them.

The bottom line was finding someone who could be with Pops during the night. That way Pops could stay in Bristol. She could attend the hospital school, which was open to siblings of patients, and she was allowed to be in hospital during the rest of the day.

There was no one in our lives who could fulfil the role of night carer. No one.

I drifted in to unconsciousness and came to as a nurse was checking H's vitals. In that 'dreamtime', that world between sleep and awake my brain did that 'thing'. The thing when it's engaged without you realising. How amazing is that? Even when we think we are asleep our brains are still at it, still whirring away, still pumping blood and still moving our lives on.

That's it! I would have to PAY someone to look after Pops at night. People had child minders and nannies. There must be a way of finding someone for the job.

It had taken a while to get there but I had found a way forward! When you simply don't have the luxury of being able to use money as a problem solver you forget it can buy more than electricity and milk. The solution had been there all along.

I had no idea where the money would come from. I would probably have to borrow against my mortgage; but there was no price anyone could put on keeping the three of us together.

I felt this overwhelming urge to touch my son. I held his hand, felt his warm flesh and then I stroked his forehead, ran my fingers through his lush curls and sat by the bed, watching him breathe. My son. The boy doctors told me my body would be unlikely to ever have, because my hormones were out of kilter, because I had a benign brain tumour, a prolactinoma, and the drugs I'd had to take were heavy duty. How miraculous my son had a sister, a third child my body had conceived, naturally, against all the medical odds.

In peaceful moments, the dreamtime between routine and bustle and necessity, there is the chance to revel in miracles. Life is full of them and we must find them, feel them and hang on for dear life. There was a way through this and whatever life had thrown, was going to throw, I'd deal with it. I had a choice. I could wash the floor with my tears or I could roll up my sleeves and get on with it.

I sat back on the plastic mattress, skin separated from stickiness by a rough cotton sheet, and resumed the pixie position. In a few months I would be taking both my children home, to our cottage and our cats. I would deal with whatever I had to in order to achieve that and I could only do it if I remained calm and focused.

One week after diagnosis and my straight jacket was still in its box.

CHAPTER TWENTY

SUNDAY WAS FILLED WITH DRUGS, CLEAN SHEETS AND A VISIT.

Pops wouldn't leave my lap; the traumas of another night spent apart taking their toll, along with the swine flu. Chris looked tired as well.

Lovely Nurse Rachel, true to her word, ushered in Doctor Helen at some point early afternoon – though consultants are called 'Mr' not 'Doctor'. Did that make Helen 'Mrs'?

'Mrs' Helen sat on the spare chair and listened, throwing in the odd question. She told me she was a mother of three, which explained the slightly care-worn, softer attire in contrast with the crisp, ironed, no nonsense lines of some other women doctors we'd met.

She said there was not much she could do, but she would talk to some people. I felt she got the message. I felt no one was connecting up the dots of our situation. Was her surprise genuine, to come across a family with our set up and resultant dilemma – one mum, two children, no family back up?

At one point she got very indignant on our account.

'Well, if anyone tells you, you can't go and buy your son a kiwi fruit, I'll go and buy him one myself,' she said.

I also shared another concern; well, I shared an awful lot of concerns. I tried very hard not to rant. When, at around lunchtime, a woman I'd never seen before carried in a tray of food for H, she removed it when I told her he wouldn't eat it, but maybe I could give it to his sister.

Doh! I hear you say. Just keep your mouth shut Sharon. Surely you must realise by now I'm not very good at that.

'We're only allowed to feed the patient,' she said, before whisking away the congealing pile of brown stuff, almost losing a limp carrot in the process.

'If I'm not allowed to leave the room Helen, how can I feed my daughter?' I said.

After a pause she told me, in her view, I was allowed to leave the room, as long as I avoided contact with anyone, wherever possible, wore a mask and tried not to cough or sneeze around other people.

I wanted to ask where I could purchase a t-shirt emblazoned with the word *unclean*.

By the time 'Mrs' Helen left, I believed progress had been made, even if she only mentioned our situation to one other person over a coffee, at least it gave more of a chance someone, somewhere, would 'get it'.

'You know what this means?' said Chris.

I looked at her, blankly.

'You can leave the hospital. There's a Tesco Express near here.'

Leave Room 4? Oh my days! Leave the room. Leave the room!???

'I can't! What about H? I can't.'

'You can,' said Chris, 'and I will sit with him. With them both. You need to do this.'

And she was, of course, absolutely right. I didn't have a time slot in my life to develop agoraphobia. Any-phobia actually.

As if planning for an arctic expedition, I set out on *Mission*

Kiwi. Feeling like an escaped convict, without *anyone on the outside,* I eventually prised myself out of the cell – I mean hospital room – and walked the long corridor, past the empty nurse's station, all the while resisting the urge to hug the wall with my back while looking left and right, left and right, checking for sentries, arms spread, feeling my way in the semi darkness, which in reality was bright strip lighting.

I made it as far as the parents' kitchen, which was empty, and turned the corner, walking the few steps to the door of Ward 34.

Despite full and proper directions from Chris as to how to 'escape', I still got lost along corridors, eventually found some stairs and headed down, all the while trying not to cough, sneeze or brush past anyone. If there had been anyone around, I'm sure they would have given me some very odd looks. I was behaving very strangely.

Normally I'm all for new experiences, new places, discovering somewhere new. *'India with no return ticket, why not? Yeah, I'll drive a truck to the Ukraine, in February. Course I can drive the car out to Italy with a five-year old map reader. Move two hundred miles to a strange town – no problem'.*

That particular Sunday I was having difficulty walking down five sets of stairs and turning right out of an enormous pair of automatic glass doors onto a pavement. It was almost as if I could see my marbles rolling off down the hill, never to be seen again.

It was dusk. I knew the sun was getting low even though it was obscured by buildings. The chill, as my face met the outside, was distinctly crisp; my cotton jacket not fit for a cold November day. I never have been very good at packing in a hurry.

I didn't like the sensation of walking away from both my children. But if H wanted a kiwi then I had to leave the hospital. And Chris was right, I needed to do this. I needed to remind myself there was a world outside the hospital. I had to remain connected, not let Room 4 become my horizon. Our horizon.

I found the said express food outlet. Like a thunderbolt between the eyes, I clocked all the Christmas marketing: A stand of special offer gold coins, chocolate advent calendars stacked high, mince pies, nets of nuts, festive Toblerone, jars of cranberry sauce-in-your-face festive demands to consume Christmas-in-your-face-no-escape.

How on earth was I going to 'do' Christmas for my children, while living in a hospital room?

Oh no – what about all the *stocking fillers* and festive treats I'd already started buying – the ones stashed in secret places and cunning hidey holes, at home, in Devon? Then the inevitable thought! What if? What if H...

Shocked at my own thought, I stood on the pavement as if I'd been winded. No imagining the funny looks I was getting.

'MOVE!' said voice in head. *'Move along. Blend in. Be like everyone else. Don't draw attention to yourself. Think kiwi.'*

So I did. Only to discover this particular outlet didn't have any to sell.

Walking up the hill towards the hospital I felt wretched. The only thing my son had wanted was a piece of kiwi fruit. And what had I managed? A fresh half cucumber. Plus a small pot of Vaseline for his dry lips, more Paracetamol, some minty chewing gum and a buy one get one free bag of gold foil chocolate coins, to go in the toes of two Christmas stockings lurking in a box somewhere in my Devon loft. And I managed a lettuce and a pot of cheddar cheese sandwich filling, no bread; I can only think the cheese addict in me had woken up but got the urge a bit topsy-turvy.

I had also managed far too many odd looks – or so I felt. Good to know paranoia was setting in. By the time I'd made it back to the fifth-floor door of Ward 34, buzzed my way in and slathered my hands in antibacterial hand gel, which I was already learning to detest because it left behind such an unpleasant sticky residue after several slatherings, I was freezing cold and felt completely useless. Sent out on safari I'd probably come back with a broken rattan chair, and an empty bottle of gin.

H did try and eat a bit of cucumber, possibly two calories worth. He was very understanding about the kiwi scenario. I promised to try harder next time. Pops failed to even smell the chocolate lurking in my handbag. She must still be in the grip of swine flu. I knew how she felt.

At least I had heard Cousin Debbie – saviour Cousin Debbie – was arriving tomorrow. I would miss Chris, but she had to get back to her own life and family.

That night, as Pops lay tucked up in the hotel room with Chris, and H was tick tick ticking and click click clicking away, I lay down, wanting the oblivion of sleep. It turned its back on me, like a disgruntled lover.

I wondered what it would be like to be here in Bristol, with a husband, a father, a partner. Easier... and harder. With only one set of emotions I couldn't argue with anyone, like I'd heard a couple earlier. But I would get a hug. I would be able to share the fear, the practicalities, know Pops was with family. Families: how complex they are.

I have often heard it said –and there are fridge magnets out there to prove it – that friends are the family of the 21st century. *God gave you your family, thank God you can choose your friends.*

Friends had already begun to send cards, letters, notes as well as calling and texting. People were offering help and their kindness, their offers, were all so well meant. But I was beginning to feel like I was flying a stricken plane, with no instruction manual and too many co-pilots to fit in the cockpit.

My head was crowded out. But it was also incredibly humbling, knowing how many people wanted to help. I was having to learn to accept help. It was not something I was very good at really.

There were schemes building out there for Pops to live in

Devon during the week, carry on with school and her friends, and get driven to Bristol each weekend. Someone could stay with her at the weekend, someone could drive her back to somewhere else on the Sunday. People were offering to do a rota, for her to spend time in Reading as well as Devon.

Another bout of tears. I knew Pops would not cope with being parcelled around and I knew H needed her in Bristol. So did I. My wider family scenario was tricky enough. I knew I had to hold on to the reigns, be the matriarch for us three. It was me who would have to pick up the pieces after all this, just as I'd had to keep applying the glue up until now. This was our life. Too many people were making suggestions, without understanding the reality of H's cancer, our situation. It was a struggle for me. People were being so kind. It was getting exhausting saying 'no thank you, that won't work because...' Was I being ungrateful, saying 'no' so often?

It deepened my resolve. The best way forward was to pay someone to care for Pops. That way there could be no misunderstandings, no embarrassments. I also felt when we got home, we wouldn't be quite so heavily burdened with the weight of feeling in so much emotional debt.

But if a friend had offered to deliver some kiwi fruit at that moment, I would have accepted, gratefully. Except we didn't know a soul in Bristol. And I couldn't ask anyone to drive up a kiwi from Devon, or down from Reading. In the world of ridiculous that would have been plain daft.

Yet we were in the world of daft. Dangerously daft. One mum. Two children. No home. Not allowed to sleep in the same place. Tears before, during and after bedtime. And not just Pops' tears.

CHAPTER TWENTY-ONE

SAYING GOODBYE TO CHRIS MEANT SAYING HELLO TO COUSIN DEBBIE, who, I realised just before she was due to arrive, I really didn't know very well.

Family gatherings were one thing - parties, weddings, funerals – but to spend time in a confined space with a relative you have 'known' all your life, yet not 'known' at all, was a new one on me.

I knew she was a hard-working, sensible and caring person. I knew she smoked and had a talent for interior design. What else did I know? Erm...

It transpired Debbie was also a coffee drinker. I realised I hadn't drunk coffee for days. Soon large cardboard cups with plastic lids started arriving, from one of the funky coffee shops which could be seen from Room 4's window.

Wearing a mask, apron and gloves was an adjustment, and a big ask for a *woman of a certain age*. I was so grateful Debbie, after a phone call, had dropped everything to help. She had called me before setting off, to try and get a measure of the situation. No doubt I had only been capable of burbling.

'Have you had a swine flu jab?' I managed to ask. The hospital was insisting she would have to have one.

Room 4 was a shocking environment to enter. I probably looked like some kind of wild woman. On a stage, my props would surely have included a carrier bag labelled kiwis and cucumbers. My children would have been playing ghosts, no need for white sheets.

Still, at least someone had been able to give me a telephone number for the phone in Room 4, which had been little more than a window sill ornament so far. It could only accept incoming calls but it gave us a connection to the outside. It didn't take long before it became intrusive. People began asking *when* was a good time to call? A number of 'well, there isn't really *a good time*' wasn't very helpful on my part. It wasn't possible to anticipate the onset of projectile vomiting or an essential sheet change. No one could know when I was talking to a doctor, or a nurse was administering. In the end I had to unplug the phone; it seemed to ring every time H nodded off.

'What you need is a blog,' said my friend and writing buddy Kate. 'Then you update everyone on line and people don't have to keep ringing.'

'But Kate, I need a computer for that, don't I?'

My writing friend, who was also an international business woman, was well used to my dismal technical failings. She also knew I refused to Facebook.

'Yes Sharon,' she said, the *'I'm being very patient with you'* tone in her voice a reassuring familiarity. 'You're going to need a laptop.'

At last, here was something positive I could ask for help with. A few phone calls later and dad had agreed to fund a laptop, despite mum's, 'How much do they cost? That much!?' in the background.

Neighbour Becky, Devon friend Julie and her Techy Husband

Richard (what would I ever have done without other people's Techy Husbands?) took up the mantle and commenced *operation laptop*. Kate fixed a visit so she could help me 'set up' the laptop, words which made me feel distinctly uneasy. Give me a needle and thread, I know where I am with that. But a portable computer with intels and giggy wotsits and multi-gesture touchpads and stuff. Weren't my synapses already under enough pressure?

They were all right though. A laptop also meant I could carry on working and write the blog. It would also key H and Pops into the world, help them with schoolwork. I'm no Luddite – hell, I've been using telephone answer machines and microwaves for years. The transition from videos to DVDs was a synch. I even know what to do with Scart sockets. But a laptop. Yes, yes, I have a computer at home, I'm not that dim. I couldn't work without one, of course I couldn't. But a laptop, writing a blog, no Techy Partner, let loose in such a world who knows where I'd end up.

You can laugh, but I have a track record. I can get computers doing things everyone says is impossible. I've had grown men – Techy Husbands, even a Techy Partner once - sitting at my screen, scratching their heads, saying 'but that's just not possible!'. I'm on first name terms with my server provider, he's called Steve. In fact, they've probably written part of their training manual around me, *what to do with the client who defies all logic.*

But at least I felt I could begin to make sense of our situation, involve H and Pops in something. It was a way of not feeling quite so isolated.

By the time Pops and Cousin Debbie had departed for the hotel, to yet another room because hotel staff were unable to book the same room on consecutive nights (incompetence or rules?), I heard a meeting had been set up with some of the hospital bureaucrats, so see if they could help us. It was a Hallelujah! moment. Who had 'Mrs' Helen spoken to?

It was a relief to think people might listen, but what did I do now? How could I explain our situation? What could they do to help? Maybe they would know how to find a paid carer? There must have been families like us through here before. We couldn't be the first, they must have helped other people like us, surely? I felt nervous, but I had to retain my focus.

I also had to keep in mind this was a hospital, here to cure H, not a facility for the dispossessed, even though it was the leukaemia which had tossed us here. I did appreciate and fully understand that.

However, I also felt the bureaucrats were being inflexible. A small mattress for Pops would solve all the practical problems, allow us to focus on getting H well. It was also the cheapest and most practical option there was at that moment in time. I found it very hard to understand why the management ethos of a children's cancer ward was unable to deal with such obvious issues faced by families who have been ripped out of their lives.

Wondering if there was any useful information in the CLIC Sargent Filofax Social Worker Lin had given me, I flicked through a few pages. There was a section entitled

'Do you have any advice for grandparents, family and friends?'

With increasing frustration, I read a list of things *'you might consider doing to help'*, which included, *shopping; school runs and after school care looking after or helping with the other children in the house; giving the carer a break and sitting with the sick child; doing the washing up or any other domestic tasks; listening – sometimes your family member/friend may value having someone to talk to; join a support group so you can find out how others in your situation have coped'.*

It was certainly a laugh or cry experience. I just laughed quietly, to myself. I may as well have been reading an advice booklet written for lone women ferret keepers in the Yemen.

Whoever had written the 'advice' had clearly not been briefed about people like us. People whose children had cancer which could not be treated at their local hospital. People who were uprooted from their homes, removed from their support networks, friends, families, the corner Co-op. There was certainly no concept of that challenging creature 'The Single Mother'. I had no kitchen sink in which to leave any washing up for someone else to do. I didn't even have a coffee mug, although I did have a 'Yellow Beryl'.

I turned for solace to the cheery booklet '*Childhood Acute Myeloid Leukaemia (AML)*'. There was a section on '*Coping with Childhood leukaemia ... advice to try and help you as a family cope with the stresses and problems of having a child with leukaemia*'.

Apart from the fact they had conveniently bi-passed the concept of 'one-parent families', I found most of what was written so patronising I wanted to burn it. Luckily, I'm not an arsonist, though I do love open fires and fireworks.

'*You have recently suffered a very severe shock because you have learned that your child has leukaemia... Now that you know the truth you are besieged by many bewildering thoughts and feelings. It is important for you to know that this is natural and that you are not unusual in having these thoughts.*'

It gets better!

'*It is hard at first not to be very depressed or angry about the news but you must remember that so much can be done today for children with leukaemia and you must have hope. Children have as good as a (sic) 70% chance of treatment being successful and these children will go on to lead completely normal lives... No one knows at the time of diagnosis which children will survive.*'

By the time I got to:

'*While it will sound very complicated and frightening to you, remember that the doctors and nurses are carrying out these treatments every day and for them it is as much routine as it is, for example, a policeman to direct traffic... The people treating your child are experts in their field. While this should give you confidence it may also make you feel inadequate.'*

I was stunned.

'Remember that you are very important to your child'... prompted me to feel the person who had written this drivel was indeed the work experience author of 'The Lone Woman's Guide to Keeping Ferrets in the Yemen'.

Under, *'Visiting and living in hospital with your child'* the guidance notes had very obviously been written with no reference to AML itself, despite the title of the booklet. The advice was so general it was useless.

For example: *'parents can come (to hospital) at any time and stay until the evening. Obviously the nurses have to settle the young in their beds and cots in the early evening, but they will encourage you to see your child settled and it is best to follow your usual routine... The ward sister will however usually allow brothers and sisters to visit at weekends and this is important so that the family can get together'.*

Well, that one was clearly written by the Victorians! By the time I read:

'Parents have a great need to talk with each other about this shock which has struck the family and to discuss their feelings, reactions and worries. You both need comfort and support and it is easier to give this to each other if you have time alone together'. It was clear I had vacated my previous universe.

'With a disease like leukaemia the ongoing treatment, although mostly on an outpatient basis, will last for months and it is important from the outset to work out a method for your family so that no one feels neglected or put upon.'

This little gem was a direct contradiction to what I had been told. H would be an in-patient for many months. The badly written advice in the patronising booklet was pathetic and I could not believe anyone in H's care team had actually read it. I'll skip over the sexist bits. It was a dangerously misleading source of information. It was the only information I had been given and I had no access to anything else. It was astonishingly awful.

Adding to the sense of ridiculousness was;

'No one will think the less of you for spending some time away from your child. We all need some time to ourselves especially at periods like this when we need to "refuel". The staff all realise how stressful it is to be on a busy ward for long hours with little to do yourself'.

Look. I'm a writer. I wrote an essay at the age of five which proclaimed, 'When I Grow up I want to be a Arthur'. Fortunately for journalism, my spelling and grammar have improved immensely. I was horrified by what I had just read. I was disgusted it had been commissioned, passed, printed, paid for and given out to parents who needed help, support and information.

I would have to find ways of being heard. At the meeting arranged for the following day I would have to not just be heard; I would have to make sure people actually listened.

I was in a minority of minorities, sub section C in an addendum which didn't appear on the index. To be listened to, I was going to have speak loudly, without raising my voice; with a throat so sore it felt like I'd swallowed a Yemeni ferret.

Wonder what Yemen's like at this time of the year?

CHAPTER TWENTY-TWO

Nurse Rachel came to get me at some point on the Tuesday. She took me up to level seven, the top floor of the hospital. I was mindful not to cough or sneeze at any point. By the time the door opened on a large room my mouth was so dry I wondered if I'd be able to talk at all.

I was offered a chair, padded with grey scratchy fabric, a square seat welded on to a metal frame. It was a change from institutional turquoise and signalled I was now in the land of bureaucrats, not clinicians; from syringe filling to pen pushing in one easy chair move.

There was no mistaking the officialdom. I found myself facing a row of six people. I knew three of them – Doctor John (consultant), Jamie (leukaemia nurse specialist) and Lin (CLIC social worker). The head of nursing and the chief matron joined them. Along with a senior administrator, who took notes and produced some rather inaccurate minutes.

I formed the opinion, unfairly or otherwise, that the note taker, however senior her title proclaimed her to be, was the kind of woman who had an accent wall in the living room papered with B&Q wallpaper; all set off by chain store cushions first spotted in a Sunday supplement. She was smart, probably hard-working and may have strayed as far as Lanzarote on a package deal. But she exhibited little life experience. The resultant notes nodded towards a sheltered view on the world. I'm sure she must have been in league with the writer of the laughable AML booklet.

Taken from the hospital's own summary of the meeting – formally entitled,

"Meeting to discuss care of H … and support that could be offered to his family – 24th November 2009.

Everyone in the room apologised for any inflexibility that the hospital had shown in dealing with this unique situation," said the notes.

It was a relief just to get some acknowledgement. It did feel like they were trying to help. Doctor John outlined the care H would need – four courses of chemo which was likely to take anything up to six months, infections during each cycle, time out for a few days between each one when we could, all three, stay at CLIC House. But for five weeks of each cycle H *"could potentially be very sick".*

The language surrounding cancer is vague. It has to be. Words like *potential, expect, may take longer, unsure how long this will take, possibilities, worst case scenario;* no one, not even the most senior of experts, could predict the course H's leukaemia would take. It made putting a care diary in place very challenging for everyone involved. I had, of course, left my crystal ball in Devon.

The swine flu remained an issue – was that why everyone was sitting so far away from me? It felt like a high-powered job interview. My social skills were being tested, my ability to perform under pressure, to articulate, make out I was a grown up in control. Forgot my CV of life. Mouth so dry. At least my attire would have impressed a field of scarecrows. I gave my litany about our situation. People seemed to be listening.

Doctor John made it very clear there would times during H's care when Pops could not stay with us. If he was admitted to PICU (Paediatric Intensive Care Unit; OMG!), for example. Or if H was very sick on the ward. Err, what had she experienced already? (I didn't say that bit out loud, obviously).

In the hospital notes I had apparently agreed H could be left on his own at night when he was well. My recollection of that is at odds with what was written down. In fact, I refute it. I had promised my son I would be with him all the way, which meant not leaving him alone at night. Wished I'd been taking my own notes.

At no point in the hospital's notes had it stated I was a single parent, the sole carer of two children.

What the notes actually said was (sic)

"Another scenario discussed is if a single parent gets sick & what support we can offer. The social work team can put something in place to support the above scenario but also if H was very sick and no carer was available. All agreed that this would only be used in the worst-case scenario".

Having swine flu, despite it then being the most fashionable disease in England, didn't count then?

There were positives to come out of the meeting. A place called *Charly's House* was offered, from the following day, as a place for us to stay. CLIC House would become a possibility when Pops and I were clear of swine flu. It was a place where we could not only stay, but there was support on offer, mainly from other uprooted families. It sounded like an oasis. It was dubbed 'a home from home'.

In short Jamie agreed to go through a possible diary of when H was most likely to be sick, which gave me a fighting chance of putting a care package together. I agreed with the bigwigs to,

"communicate in advance where there is a gap in her care schedule."

The notes were wrapped up with,

"All agreed that the default position is that Pops does not stay but exceptional circumstances will be discussed when they arise with the hospital agreeing to be flexible".

Despite the inaccuracy of the notes – which even suggested H could be treated in Exeter, despite every doctor denying they had the facilities to do so - there was definite progress. Obviously, I couldn't tell hospital management that my entire care schedule was, currently, one huge gap. I also had yet to find a way of paying someone to care for Pops.

The hospital could not suggest where I might look for a paid carer. But I would have a piece of paper stating Pops was, SOMETIMES, allowed to stay in hospital overnight. It could be used as a weapon in the future, if any more Nasty Nurses chose to cross my tolerance threshold, which by then was thinner than a cat's whisker. The cats! What on earth was I going to do about the cats? Friends couldn't feed them indefinitely and Ruby really needed company. She was still a kitten.

Snapping back to reality – whatever that was - Jamie and Lin were now fully in the picture and I really felt they were on my side, despite there being no actual solution to our situation. I had to put my faith in them. I felt they could both be trusted.

'I have no money to pay a carer,' I confessed to them both. There would be a way, they both said. Did that mean they could help?

Lin said she would look into grants. She had never come across a family in our situation before. The closest she could recall was a Cornish family with three children who ran a pub, which was also their home. One parent came to Bristol to care for the sick child while the other stayed in Cornwall to look after the remaining two. Except the parent left in Cornwall could not care for both the remaining children, and run the pub. If they didn't run the pub, they all lost their home.

The solution had been to fund a nanny. The family had paid a third and two other charities had paid the remainder. Lin thought she might be able to find a charity which could help us.

I found it very hard to believe we were the first single parent family, with no back up, Bristol Children's Hospital had ever encountered. But then again, we were now in a very elite group of people. We'd hit a childhood cancer *sub group*. It was called AML.

Of the ten families a day who are told their child has cancer, many can be treated closer to home, certainly as out-patients after they are stabilised. Not many cancers required up to six months as an in-patient. AML was not just aggressive; it was rare in children.

If we'd had to cope for a couple of weeks, even a month, we could have muddled through. We were expert muddlers. But six months? Tough for a two-parent family, where one or both parents work. It was Doctor John who had described our situation as a *Perfect Storm*. I could almost feel the hail slashing at my face.

Clutching a handful of invisible straws, I followed Rachel back to ward 34. She had been sitting on a chair by a wall throughout the meeting. It must have been then I properly saw her face. Don't sneeze, I thought. She was really pretty, quite young, pale skinned. It must have been incredibly intimidating for her, the meeting, being faced with a raft of her own bosses.

Then it struck me. Despite my Saharan mouth I had spoken up, articulated my position, not agreed with everything. I had made headway. I had set a precedent. Pops WAS allowed to stay in hospital overnight, sometimes. And actually, they were right on one point. It wasn't the best environment for Pops. But I maintained it was better for her to stay in Bristol and that had been supported by Doctor John. Pops was officially part of H's 'Get Well' plan. He needed her in Bristol, and that was the view of doctors.

Now it was official. Pops was staying in Bristol, no matter what anyone thought.

Clichés are terribly bad for us writers, but all I could think was *where there's a will, there's a way.*

I had the will. Now, where was the way?

CHAPTER TWENTY-THREE

The meeting gave a bit of excitement to take back to Room 4. Charly's House. No more anonymous hotel rooms.

Pops would be able to feel we had our own space and it would be easier for Debbie. It meant we'd have a fridge again. And wardrobes. Debbie had a 'thing' about cardigans and she had some beautiful ones. They needed hangers, not a suitcase.

Charly's House was another charity property, at the disposal of the bone marrow unit. It was a solution for a family ridden with swine flu. And cancer. It was available.

Someone told me it was closer than CLIC House and had been recently re-furbished. Apparently, it was a rather nice three storey town house filled with brand new Next furniture. It would certainly be different from our Devon cottage.

First the property had to be deep cleaned, which was a relief. At some point someone, from somewhere, dropped Charly's House door keys in to Room 4. It was a welcome distraction for Debbie and Pops. It meant they could move in the following day.

I gave Debbie some money. I didn't want her to be out of pocket in Bristol and it meant she would be able to buy food, stock up the fridge!

It was also becoming apparent Pops needed all sorts of things. I had packed in such a hurry; neither of the children had many out of school clothes because they wore uniforms. It didn't take long for the limitations of Pops' wardrobe to shine through, particularly as it was beginning to get very cold. I'm always a bit slow preparing for winter. My usual reluctance to let go autumn days of gold, the kind which glow with low sky sun and hum with fruity promise, would be waning if we were home in Devon. Here in Bristol being ill equipped was down to lack of resources, not because I was hanging on to memories of summer warmth and hot sand.

Debbie whisked Pops off shopping – much to her horror, shopping was not my daughter's favourite pastime – and she was soon sporting a black and neon pink striped hat and scarf from a well know high street store, dubbed by hospital staff *'Primani'*. In the land of the dispossessed it was a shining star. From pyjamas to blankets, quilt covers to mugs and shower mats you could furnish a hospital room inside a couple of large brown paper carrier bags for less than it would cost for a ticket to the theatre.

Tuesday blended into Wednesday. H was still on chemo; Pops was still a lost soul and I still could not stop crying at every given private moment. Debbie was a rock, simply getting on with it.

By then we also had Blutac. The room no longer looked so clinical. When cards arrived, I stuck them on the walls. Becky had posted photographs of the cats and chickens, which Pops and I pinned up. It was an incredibly kind and thoughtful gesture. It was also a form of *extreme nesting*, a type of *displacement therapy*, for the abandoned. Hospital staff were very tolerant.

My friend Kate came to visit on the way back from a business meeting in Stratford; we talked computers. She'd set up a blog and a new email address using our *crazy blood* tag line, which summed up the entire scenario.

Debbie and Pops returned from Charly's House, full of how big it was.

We now had access to a three-storey town house with a huge TV so complicated I'd probably not be able to switch it on. It also had a very large boiler with a complicated control panel – apparently designed for high spec robots.

The property was Georgian and clearly had, at one point, been a grand and elegant house. It's 21st century incarnation had three bedrooms, three bathrooms, a large living room to house the enormous TV, a second living room/playroom, an under stair cupboard which I later discovered seemed to have a similar floor area to Room 4, a dining room with a second TV, a front door, a back door leading on to a courtyard larger than our Devon garden.

Pops was animated, talking about Charly's House. The back entrance hallway, sporting many handy coat hooks, had a second inner door leading into a fully equipped kitchen/diner. I had always dreamed of having a kitchen diner! Next to the downstairs loo was a person height cupboard, housing a nearly new washer drier. On the top floor was a huge walk-in airing cupboard, racked out and stacked with supplies of huge brown towels and beige bedding. All from Next. I felt sure in days past it had been stacked with pure white cotton tablecloths, edged with handmade lace, spotless linen napkins and Egyptian white sheets ironed to perfection using nothing more than hissing hot metal.

It all seemed so incredibly excessive when all we'd needed, or wanted, was a small child's mattress so Pops could sleep in Room 4.

Within 24 hours Debbie and Pops also discovered you couldn't get hot water in the kitchen, the boiler had just the two settings – on boiling hot or off – and you couldn't use the microwave because they had to wedge it up against the kitchen tap as it was dripping so badly it was virtually a gush. There was no point using the dishwasher either, because there simply weren't enough plates, cups, teaspoons, knives, bowls or essentials to stack before you ran out and could justify turning it on. Boiling a kettle to wash up was easier.

During their first evening in the house, the Wednesday night, Debbie and Pops also discovered several piles of congealed rice and, what had possibly once been 'egg foo young', gluing themselves to both a posh Next table and the nearly new neutral carpet. So much for a deep clean in a house usually set up to accommodate people who had just had a bone marrow transplant, people who had virtually no immunity.

By the Thursday morning I was trying to find out who was responsible for the running of the house. We needed someone to come and fix the kitchen tap and the boiler. There was a choice between having no heat at all, or the house being so hot you had to open the windows to let the cold air flood in on a regular basis. Boiling hot bedrooms and hormonal surges did not sit together, as Debbie had already found out.

Messages were left with people. No one called back. As situations of the barking variety went, it was ridiculous in the extreme. I found it hard enough to keep up with maintenance in my own home – the one abandoned in Devon – and now I was also responsible for a three-storey town house in a strange city with a knackered boiler and a tap leaking so badly it probably needed its own water bill.

I sound so ungrateful. Being handed the keys to such a lovely property. I was, however, extremely grateful as it had given Pops a distraction and, I hoped, made it a bit easier for Debbie. But how many sponsored walks or London balls would it take to pay the gas bill?

Thursday brought a visit from two Devon friends, Hayley and Julie, who arrived in Room 4, laden with bags of goodies from well-wishers in Devon. They had already had a huge bunch of flowers confiscated before even getting into the lift. It was learning curve stuff; no plants were allowed on the ward as they were an infection risk to patients. Apparently, bacteria lurk in the water and spores can cause all sorts of damage.

The shock waves surrounding H's diagnosis had travelled far. People I barely knew sent things – sweets, comics, cards, chocolate, chocolates, teddies, craft kits, Meccano, books, funky pens. Alongside a growing chocolate mountain was wine, from Hayley's own 'cellars'.

'Oh Hayley, I can't!' I said. 'It's a dry ward.' Her face fell. I realised I'd not had a drink for days and days.

'I'll leave you with it,' she said, 'you'll need a drink soon!' The moment came sooner than anticipated.

Room 4 was getting too crowded. Debbie and Hayley decided I needed a break from its confines and frog marched me out towards a wine bar type pub that could be seen from the window of our 'cell'. Julie stayed with H and Pops.

We got in the lift and in it was a woman suffering a clear case of *talking disease*. Without knowing me from Eve she wittered on about how she'd had to stay in hospital for a while but the weeks went really quickly and before she knew it, she was home. I must have looked in need of some comfort.

'Weeks?' I said, through heavily gritted teeth. 'For us its months!'

'Oh that'll soon pass dear,' she said, as Hayley and Debbie escorted me – yes, physically, from the lift. I think they must have seen the volcano about to erupt. It was quelled with red wine, swiftly administered, while I must have burbled for England, all the while sitting within sight of Room 4's window.

Of course, drinking two glasses of red wine, large, wasn't sensible. My head was floating anyway. Plans were bandied about. It was helpful to have other view points and talking away from the hospital environment seemed to offer greater clarity – or was that red wine thinking? Everything felt unreal. Was this bar a figment of my imagination? Was the bar real and Room 4 an illusion, my son's cancer an aberration? Everything out here seemed so *'normal'*. People were sitting at tables, talking to each other, buying drinks, flirting with the bar maid. A Bristol events magazine proved there was a whole world outside of Room 4. I could feel the energy around me, the room was buzzing with life. The contrast of the environments - trendy bar versus Room 4 – could not have been greater. It left me feeling surreal, untethered to anything, adrift in a sea of emotions so intense I wanted to be shipwrecked.

Fortunately I was tethered, by an astronaut's oxygen line, the need to be near both my children so powerful if I hadn't gone back when I did, I'm not sure I would have been able to carry on breathing.

By the time we were back in Room 4 – with no further incidents, lift or otherwise - I felt like I'd had a week's holiday, such was the intensity of our situation. Maybe we should be pioneering change of environment mini breaks – so much greener, don't you think?

Julie and Hayley had to drive back to Devon to pick up children from school. Their visit meant so /much. I didn't feel quite so isolated; yet I still felt very alone. Hayley was one of the funniest women I knew, and we did laugh that day. I had so needed that; it was like a safety valve. I suspect Debbie had needed it too. But as both my friends were returning to their own lives, ours felt even more lost.

I knew I was out of sorts because in Room 4 were three rather lovely bottles of wine, stashed in a bag in the corner, and I didn't have even the tiniest urge to open one. And it was nothing to do with not having a glass with a stem.

CHAPTER TWENTY-FOUR

THE NEXT FEW DAYS BLURRED INTO EACH OTHER, AS IF ROOM 4 WAS A satellite orbiting our previous existence.

I was able to start putting together a 'care diary' for Pops. Chris had set the ball rolling and now the CLIC Filofax was filling with names scrawled across dates. The world turned. High sided blue trays continued appearing. Sheets were changed. H was off oxygen. The room felt cold.

Pops had started at the hospital school, though the Friday morning had not got off to a great start.

The hospital's own never before heard from *Secret Sub-Committee Dealing with Swine Flu*, had been convened in a broom cupboard somewhere. It had been decreed Pops, myself and Debbie were, indeed, officially allowed to leave Room 4 if we wore a mask until we got outside the big glass hospital doors, the ones which led to 'The Outside'.

On the Friday morning, just as Pops was about to charge through the door into Room 4 for a big mummy hug, someone stopped her. It was all a bit dramatic, almost a physical portrayal of seeing her taken away from me.

I pressed the red button, demanded to know what was

happening. I opened the door, stepped out of Room 4 into the corridor – mask-less – still demanding to know what was happening. Someone was trying to steal my daughter. I had to stop them! The scene would have been a wrap in one click of the clapperboard.

Someone told me to get back in the room. I refused until someone told me what was happening. Debbie hung on to Pops, both of them rabbits in headlights.

I think Pops had been waiting all night for a hug from me just as I had been up most of the night needing to cuddle my daughter. We had been seconds away from touching. As the tears broke through, I started shouting for someone to tell me what the hell was going on, at the same time telling Pops not to worry, mummy would sort it out.

Amid the confusion Debbie took Pops away to the school as I told my daughter to go, everything would be alright. They walked away, Pops looking back all the while, her face etched with a BAFTA award-winning look of abject misery.

Out of the needless drama came an eventual explanation.

The *Swine Flu Broom Cupboard Committee* had come to the conclusion Pops and I posed a risk. Yes, I know. Words failed me too. Our very clothes could have contaminated other people. Well, yes, they could have from the moment we arrived. ACTUALLY!

A school teacher had received a message from someone, somewhere – no one was sure who – saying if Pops wanted to attend school, she couldn't go into Room 4 to see H before attending class, unless she changed all her clothes before arriving in the hospital schoolroom.

It made sense. Other patients' safety was paramount. What didn't make sense was taking twelve days to come to this conclusion. The words 'horse', 'gate' and 'bolted' were beyond cliché appropriate.

Not only was the advice, however sensible, far too late but no one had communicated it to the people who really needed to know. Like the nurses on duty or the matron - who did exist – and least of all me or Debbie.

The poor schoolteacher, who most likely assumed everyone else had been told, was simply doing his job. Instead, he was faced with a hysterical mother throwing a hissy fit, a distressed child and a number of confused hospital staff failing to calm the situation because they had no idea what was going on. No doubt other angst-ridden parents of children fighting cancer were also pretty unsettled, by then the very mention of *swine flu* enough to cause terror.

I was furious. How was it possible for the hospital rule makers, whichever *subcommittee* was involved, to fail so spectacularly, to communicate something so important? And why had it taken them so long to discuss a life-threatening scenario playing out at the heart of the very hospital they were paid to manage. They were almost two weeks behind the curve.

I have always held store by the sentiment (cliché?) *fail to prepare and you prepare to fail. Fail to communicate,* declares my own version, *and no one will listen.*

I fully appreciated the precautions. It was essential to stop the spread of swine flu. But I was beginning to feel the management structures within Bristol Children's Hospital was so lumbering they could only fail.

I had no difficulty appreciating why swine flu had morphed into such horror headlines. It was, by November 2009, predicted tens of thousands would die, across the globe, from swine flu. Society as we knew it could break down. Essential workers would fall sick and die, bodies would not get buried, bins not get emptied, hospitals would overflow, the National Grid would collapse, disease would spread faster and supermarkets would be filled with gun-toting looters as supply chains ground to a halt.

I should 'fess up at this point. I believe, one day, humankind will wipe itself out with a rogue infection cooked up in a lab somewhere. I was a fan of the 1970's BBC drama, 'Survivors'.

We could indeed have been months away from the end of the world, claimed extreme headlines. Yet some idiot tucked away in a Bristol broom cupboard had failed to action a full and responsible quarantine around us three. Maybe the memo got lost on the way to the toilet. Let's hope he washed his hands. (And wised up before March 2020...)

I had increasingly begun to feel there was a ravine-shaped divide between the clinical side of the hospital, and the clerical. We had experienced how the incredible medical expertise translated into a let's get the job done, a think-on-your-feet attitude.

Immediately when the swine flu emerged, doctors had discussed the situation with me, asked for my opinion, and invited discussion. I trusted them. They made me feel as if I was as part of getting H well as they were. I deeply appreciated their approach, particularly as I'm allergic to being patronised.

It had not been apparent any of the management team had stopped to take minutes, note conclusions, issue memos or ping out emails to a carefully selected user group, which then necessitated 38 replies just to get a counter signature for the next consignment of toilet rolls. Though I did appreciate a number of office-bound signatures must have been required to authorise further supplies of latex gloves, plastic aprons and the rapidly diminishing supplies of disposable masks.

The doctors and nurses were *doing* in the present, while the managers were *talking* futures, taking days to send out missives. Now I know it's the way large organisations work – I've got letters after my name, don't you know, I have knowledge in how people and organisations and politics work together; it's called Community Studies.

I am also the great niece of a woman who spent much of her

working life as a formidable matron in and around London. Great Auntie Dot's legendary approach to nursing was often talked about at family gatherings and she was, indeed, a formidable character. There was never any doubt she was able to communicate her professionalism on every level.

I am well aware there have been many debates in recent years on the changes in the structure of the NHS. Observations on how the number of clinical staff remains fairly constant (I'm generalising) but how the number of *managers* has increased out of all proportion.

I felt we were experiencing the sharp end of those changes. That one tiny moment, when Pops was barred from Room 4, with no warning and no explanation, summed up how damaging inadequate communication can be.

We spend billions on overseas aid, billions on wars we didn't start and billions on the NHS. Yet we still live in a country where children die at the hands of their parents because teachers, police officers, health professionals and social workers don't always talk to each other. They don't talk because management structures, funding cuts, unrealistic guidelines, fear of litigation and human error are more powerful forces combined than common sense and courage. It's no surprise Hollywood favours maverick doctors, lawyers and ordinary folk who exhibit extraordinary levels of courage, by 'doing' not 'talking'.

The failures in communication at Bristol Children's Hospital, between the bureaucrats and the doers, could have caused an outbreak of swine flu inside a high dependency paediatric oncology ward.

It is a testament to the knowledge and skills of the doctors and nurses treating H that the swine flu was successfully contained within Room 4 and did not, to my knowledge, lead to another case.

After Pops arrived back from school, which only taught in the mornings, she ate a bit of the lunch which arrived for H and we headed off to Bristol city centre, leaving Debbie with H. I am not sure who was holding whose hand. I was desperate to spend some time with her. Much as she hated shopping, she needed a new coat.

It was also the plan for her to show me Charly's House. I was so proud of my seven-year-old daughter. I didn't have a clue where I was going, yet she was able to show me. Despite my little girl having swine flu she had been forced to do a fair bit of walking since we had arrived in Bristol, just twelve days previously.

She had walked to the hotel with Chris and Debbie each night and morning, into town with Debbie and round the back of the hospital to Charly's House. While I had been glued to H's bedside Pops had been our scout, our city explorer. It was Pops who had had to show other people around and now it was my turn. My biggest memory of that afternoon was the feel of my little girl's hand in mine.

As we walked, I couldn't help thinking how lucky we had been to end up at a hospital slap bang in the middle of a city centre. It soon became apparent it was a shoppers' heaven, bursting with every high street name anyone could possibly require. I'm not averse to shopping but in recent years I'd had very little opportunity, unless you counted supermarkets.

I was still finding it odd, being away from Room 4. I found it very difficult, being surrounded by the normal workings of a regular, everyday environment packed full of other people's routine stuff, just another average day, nothing out of the ordinary. Our life had become extra-ordinary, everything mundane and familiar gone. Our *usual* was nothing more than a memory.

I bought familiar soap and shampoo from Holland and Barrett. I was still persisting in the idea we should not be overloading our bodies with unnecessary chemicals. Even I could see the irony, what with H hooked up to substances which could probably kill a full-grown rhinoceros.

Pops guided me in to '*Priman*', the huge four storeys new to Bristol. We found her a coat and a long-sleeved tee-shirt. I could see she was fading.

'Let's go find a treat,' I said, and her face lit up as we discovered the M&S Food Hall. Amongst all the Christmas fare, artfully marketed, Pops was thrilled to find *Satsuma juice.*

It was beginning to get dark as we headed back up a hill towards the hospital, towards Charly's House.

I was learning Bristol is a city of hills, but nothing had quite prepared me for the hill which led directly to Pops' new *home from home.* I was surprised not to find Olympic runners training on it. Pass the oxygen. It was incredibly steep. I couldn't see the top. My thigh muscles started screaming half way up *abandon hope all ye who attempt this one.* By the time we reached the top I felt like I was in training for Everest. I also felt exceedingly shaky, despite all the time spent in the gym back home.

'We're nearly there mummy,' said Pops. 'It's quite a big hill, isn't it?'

I tried to communicate between wheezings. I wasn't going to let the hill beat me.

We turned right at the top, walked past a bohemian back street pub and there was an exclusive car park, leading to a garden gate and a mounted plaque proclaiming, 'Charly's House'. I opened the door and like excited children – well, one of us actually was a child – we stared around the freezing cold kitchen. Just as I was about to have a guided tour of the house the lights went off. In trying to find the switch I almost fell over the table.

'Don't worry love,' I said to Pops. 'I'm sure I can fix it.'

Elated I could at last show my daughter a bit of magic I found the *torch* function, which I had discovered while fiddling with my new mobile.

Just as I was figuring I could stand on a chair and get to the fuse box on the wall in the hallway, the phone rang.

It was a friend of my mum's. I knew I had to talk to her as she was pencilled in for the weekend after Debbie left, to help with Pops. By the end of the call, I just wanted to cry. There had been crossed wires. It wasn't me who had spoken to her. Her own daughter was home that weekend so she couldn't come and help. It seemed an offer of help had lost something in translation. To her it had been a thought, to a friend of mine it had been an offer.

'Terribly sorry, let me know how you're getting on...'

It wasn't her fault. It wasn't anybody's fault.

The phone rang again. Typical. There I was, standing on a chair in the dark trying to fix a fuse box and still no escape from the phone. Well, you needn't have answered it I hear you shout. But back then every phone call could have been a solution to a problem, an offer of help, a way forward.

It was my ex-mother-in-law. It was easier to answer it, make out everything was fine, than have to call her back another time.

Since she had arrived back from Spain she had been promising to come and help whenever we needed her, that she could leave sick hubby for a couple of nights if he didn't have any hospital appointments.

'Great timing,' I said. 'We really need some help weekend after next. I've just got a gap in the diary.' Actually, the diary was still more *gap* than filled.

'Oh, sorry Sharon, I can't that weekend. We're off to a do. How about the one after?'

'It's OK, I really need help the weekend before. Is there any way you could come and stay with Pops, we really need some help here?' I said, trying not to sound quite so pissed off, feeling her granddaughter was bit more important than yet another party, after a such a long holiday in the sun.

'I've already got the tickets,' she said chirpily, 'should be a good night. We're really looking forward to it.'

There I was, standing on a chair, in the dark hallway of a strange house, my daughter looking up at me waiting for the lights to go on, fortunately unable to hear a grandmother gabbling on about going to a party instead of supporting her family who, it could be said, were in pretty dire need. At least she was being true to herself. I'd known for years the word *flighty* fitted her like a glove. She was notoriously unreliable.

It seemed our default position in life, our regular, normal, everyday was simply sliding into the sewage pit. I began to wonder how long it would be until I hit the bottom.

CHAPTER
TWENTY-FIVE

DESPITE ALL THE SETBACKS, WHICH HAD TORNADOED THEIR WAY THROUGH our life in the previous two weeks, there was only one approach I could allow myself. In those dark, early days of AML I'd had to believe each hour we lived through was a step forward, even if it wasn't. Each day survived must be a day closer to taking both my children home.

Saturday, two weeks in, and an Evening Star arrived, in the shape of Lorraine. My sewing pals had made a quilt for H.

From bright primary colours each of my nimble-fingered buddies had sewn squares and then pieced them together, with vibrant accent blocks which zinged with energy and life. On the back a whizzy machine stitched label, hand stitched in place:

'*For H with love from Chris Cilla Eileen Jeannie Joan Judy Lorraine Sandra Wendy November 2009.*'

It made H smile so much I couldn't contain my tears. H's quilt came with a promise; one for Pops would follow soon. Almost immediately it became a talking point for anyone who came into the room. I was incredibly touched my friends had made something so glorious, in such a short time. They were all busy with jobs and families, houses, husbands and challenges of their own.

Let's not forget Chris had already been with us for several days, AND she was directing a play.

I knew it wasn't just the time to sew a few squares. It was the time they had taken to discuss, plan and put it all together. It was a simple quilt but stitching life into such a visual spectacular would have taken thought, skill, coordination and a matching of diaries I knew from personal experience, it was a tricky task with such a dynamic group of women.

How do you say thank you for such a wonderful thing?

My feelings that day had echoed the few words I'd pinged out on the new blog which, much to my amazement, worked. I was not for a moment suggesting I doubted my friend Kate's technical brilliance. I meant I was amazed I'd been able to press the right buttons.

In just 170 words I had communicated with the world outside Room 4. The first *Crazy Blood* Blog had finished with...

'in the meantime, we have discovered the ultimate cure for nits (hair loss, silly). So, every time I make you laugh or make you think or make you realise how special and precious your children, your family, your friends are, send H a Get Well Soon smile. If you can smile someone better then we are already well on the way.'

OK, OK I know it was schmaltzy. But back then I was wearing everything on my sleeve, including pee, pooh and vomit, though not my own I might add. Luckily the new bed adornment was fully washable.

H's quilt was a bright shining star in those dark, early days. Lorraine had brought other gifts from The Evening Stars including a miniature Christmas tree with twinkling LED lights on the end of the branches, chocolate and a funky fleece hat for H. Which reminded me, we had yet to have the *'you're-going-to-lose-all-your-hair'* conversation.

Advent Sunday came and went. Debbie and Pops were still struggling with a rogue boiler and a gushing kitchen tap but having their 'own place' was much better than a different hotel room each night.

Monday saw my next blog:

"Firstly, H is doing well. This morning (Monday November 30) finished first 10-day block of chemo. All progressing as per plan with the expected infection set in already. All perfectly 'normal' (have no idea what that word means anymore!!!) and blood cultures being grown so docs can be very specific with the antibiotics.

"Am experiencing technical difficulties ... For once it's not my idiot brain. Software on brand new laptop (bloody Windows 7) apparently faulty. Not my opinion, comes from younger brain than mine who knows about such stuff. Have considered locking second cousin Ollie in hospital room until fixed...

"Still, have acquired teacher's laptop and, as we are still in isolation because of the swine flu (two weeks plus and counting) am becoming a complete 'Borrower' and 'hanger on' to anything that comes my way...

"You have no idea of the secret leukaemia world we have entered and I hope to God no one I know or ever meet has to enter it, but layered with swine flu and the resultant isolation in a small hospital room (en suite an essential and most civilised) the world has almost found a way to silence me – I did say almost... Best hope to Goodness it's not me who gets unleashed on the computer people, cannot tell you how frustrating it is to have such amazing and clever friends who have organised, set up and trained me in the art of the laptop, only to find it's a duffer. Thanks Microsoft – not...

"But I am no longer techno-idiot, I am Crazy Blood Mum on a Mission. My Mission is to help get H better so I will beat the technology. Might add, cannot get him well without the most amazing nurses and doctors in the world, who we are lucky enough to be surrounded by in Bristol! Boy are we lucky with the oncology team here....

"With love to everyone out there. Thank you all for such tremendous support, which is manifesting itself in so many different ways. We

are privileged to have you all in our lives and look forward to catching up with all of you.

"Love Crazy Blood Mum, proud carer of H and Pops xxx"

Before I could even contemplate writing another blog, the following day brought a bombshell. H was diagnosed with a fungal infection in his lungs.

I was terrified for my son. It was something I had been dreading as I had been told by doctors it was, at that stage, a worst-case scenario. H was now fighting leukaemia, swine flu and an invasive lung fungus.

In my mind I saw the fungus as a spreading black mass of tiny spores, creeping their way around H's insides. I blame too much Doctor Who. Though in giving it a face I somehow felt it would be easier to defeat. I was so scared for H I had to turn it into a battle, with only one possible victor. I believed in both Dr John and Dr Michelle but that faith could not displace the fear. I'd thought measles was bad and both my children (and a four-year old me) had come through that one. They had surely been helped by my antibodies, imparted through a total of three years breast feeding.

Behind fear is often guilt. I had only fed H for a year because I was three months gone with Pops and no one could tell me if it was a good idea to feed while pregnant. But I was determined to make it to a year. Pops certainly didn't suffer and she was happy to feed for two years. That was the guilt. It was my fault because I'd only managed the one year for H.

Don't be daft said voice in head, masquerading as a confident Goddess. *You could not have given your son leukaemia antibodies. That's not the way this one works.* 'She' was right. So, therefore, the fungus had to be my fault, because we lived in an ancient cottage with old crevices and prehistoric spores hidden in secret landscapes behind skirting boards.

'Get a grip woman' said sensible one in head. While I was corralling my thoughts, beating the negativity out of them, the doctors were doing sensible things, like administering high end anti-fungal drugs. At one point H was being given two doses of a drug which cost £750 a time. *Fight the fear with faith*, said voice in head. Blimey, that sounded like I'd entered the world of trendy computer gaming. Except this was real. And I couldn't deny how sick I felt inside.

The phone rang.

'Yes,' I said, 'we'll see you tomorrow.'

Mum and dad were coming to see us. They would stay two nights as Debbie had to go home. Then one of my two primary school friends, Lizzie, was due on Friday for two nights. I was desperate to see her. She was an experienced senior nurse, who had turned her back on banking after nursing her mum through illness. I knew she would be able to talk me through any number of possible scenarios. We'd known each other since the days of Black Jacks and Fruit Salads, four for half a penny from the sweet shop on the way home from school.

It was overwhelming wondering how on earth I could juggle everyone. But I'd held the hoards at bay for long enough. They were going to storm the barriers whether I was ready or not. And it simply was not right to keep family away any longer.

Yet I was frightened of so many people coming through Room 4. Anxiety levels at the increased infection risk to H were rising by the hour. Now their dad was coming as well.

Hoping for a distraction I turned to the growing pile of *stuff* in the corner of the room, encased in various re-usable bags.

Among the gifts from The Evening Stars was a package from a former Reading neighbour and fellow stitcher, Sandra. More tears, when I discovered she had put together the most glorious sewing kit for me. Inside a properly partitioned plastic box was an array of basic sewing tools, from pins, needles and cotton to scissors and a thimble.

With the sewing essentials came a pile of fat quarters – a quilters term for a square quarter metre of material – plus wadding and instructions for Japanese folded patchwork, a clever technique which meant I could hand sew an entire quilt, while sitting at a hospital bedside.

It is why they had asked about H's favourite colours, to gather the right fabrics. Unfortunately, they had also asked about colours for Pops. Orange and purple are not particularly quilt friendly colours. The challenge would, I felt sure, prompt plenty of discussion...

Sewing had been my sanity after H and Pops were born, a childhood passion re-ignited. Long winter nights after the children were in bed had been filled with mad stitching sessions, gaping holes of loneliness filled with piles of fabric.

I had learnt so much from The Evening Stars. Fabric hunting excursions with Chris had given us adventures to new places. Searching out quilt shops and visiting exhibitions had given me a framework when the children were tiny, the double buggy no bar to getting through doors leading to every possible fabric-inspired opportunity.

It was now up to me whether I stitched my own straight jacket or chose to sew my way to sanity. It was thanks to Sandra, Chris and The Evening Stars I now had the means.

CHAPTER TWENTY-SIX

THE FUNGAL INFECTION INVADING H'S LUNGS HAD PROMPTED THE URGENT need for a CT scan.

I began to understand why Bristol Children's Hospital had been built on such a small footprint. It was so it could fit neatly beside the enormous Bristol Royal Infirmary. It meant paediatrics had a direct link to high spec scanning equipment, which could never have otherwise been afforded.

The appointment was confirmed, a wheelchair was found and a nurse procured. I was concerned when I heard the nurse was Loshi, a wonderfully calm, laid back and highly knowledgeable mother-of-one who was also a diabetic. I would have followed her anywhere. Except I knew the ward was so short staffed she'd not had a break and her relaxed attitude was exacerbated by increasingly obvious low blood sugar levels.

When I discovered the way to the CT scanning department was through a connecting corridor between hospitals, which took you directly through a very busy A&E department, I was concerned about the risk of infection. I was even more concerned when I asked Loshi about H's drip stand. How could we take him on such a journey, hooked up to a drip bag which led directly to his *wiggly?*

'Loshi, can't we disconnect him before we go?' I asked. 'It's not chemo. It's just a fluid.'

I was assured it would be 'fine' in a vague way but I could tell Loshi herself wasn't 'fine'. By the time we had walked out of Ward 34, Loshi pushing H's wheelchair, I was in a state of what can best be described as *high anxiety.* By the time we were approaching the A&E ward I was behaving like I was on day release from an institution and I don't mean a spa hotel. H was wearing a mask, to protect others from his swine flu. I must have been too. We were getting funny looks, Loshi was jerking the wheelchair as I was trying to keep up with her erratic movements pushing the drip stand, visions of my son's *wiggly* being yanked out of his chest building by the moment.

When I couldn't take it any longer, I shouted at Loshi to stop, telling her I'd push both. She was trying to calm me down when we were confronted by a man in blue scrubs, demanding to know what we were doing in the corridor which was, apparently, forbidden.

Being closer to exploding than crying I just managed to communicate we were trying to get my son to the CT scanning department and how was I supposed to know this wasn't the way and ...

Had I looked more closely at the time I would have realised men in shining white armour aren't always tall, dark and brooding. He was balding and kind, must have clocked my close-to-losing-it expression and calmly stepped in with an assertive 'OK, let's get you there safely, shall we.'

He pushed the wheelchair while I followed with the drip stand. I was concentrating so hard on not hurting H with an unnecessary jerk I barely noticed the route. Loshi walked alongside. I could almost feel her relief at being relieved of the responsibility of getting us there.

By the time we entered the scanning room Mr Blue Scrubs had spoken to the team in situ and told me he was going to deal with the line as it would be impossible to do the scan while H was still connected.

'Yes, thank you, I tried to tell them that back on the ward,' I said, burbling for England, 'but no one would listen and then I didn't know about the corridor and I was scared it would get yanked and I'm sorry if ...'

He held up a hand, telling me it was fine, he would sort it and, yes, he would make sure it would be OK to go back using that corridor. He was an A&E person with real authority. I wondered, what with his calm, caring attitude, if I could ask for a reassuring masculine hug? Fortunately I didn't, so I avoided making a complete fool of myself. I was feeling as wrung out as Loshi was looking. It turned out the drip was something to do with potassium and I had been right. It should have been disconnected before we had left Ward 34.

Such a tiny drama in the scheme of things. It underlined for me the pressure I was living under, trying to keep it all together, trying so desperately to do the right thing. For some reason I floated back to a life-saving swimming badge; I was a teenager, in a tatty 1920's Lido, in my growing up town. I had to tread water while making a float out of a pair of dad's old pyjamas. It was exhausting after 20 minutes but I could hear the examiner's voice from above *'come on, just another ten minutes, you can do it!'* I got the badge. Thirty odd years on and I felt like I was treading water for three lives.

Snapping back to the present Loshi and I had to walk back, she pushing the drip stand, unconnected, as I pushed my son. My neck ached from the lead jerkin the team velcroed me into when I insisted on staying in the room with H. I had promised I would be with him and, reckless or not, I had been.

Back in Room 4 Pops was with grandma and granddad. They had arrived just before we had to leave for the scan.

Mum was full of questions, dad had nodded off sitting on a plastic chair, his head lolled forwards.

'Is dad alright?' I asked mum.

'Oh he's fine. He does that all the time these days,' she said. 'Doesn't matter where he is, he just nods off.' Mum was emotional about H, but talked practicalities, like what was for dinner and which room at Charly's House could they sleep in.

Dad woke up, didn't really seem to realise where he was. He stood up, I gave him a hug. He didn't smell like my Dad. Astonishingly he'd given up smoking a week after H was diagnosed. He had smoked cigarettes since the age of 14. I'd grown up watching him roll his own, used to be sent out to buy him tins of Golden Virginia from the higgledy-piggledy newsagents, in the days when children could get away with it.

By the time my parents had moved from Berkshire to Dorset, some years previously, he had switched to a pipe. It caused just as many rows with Mum, though he had been forced to give up smoking in the toilet when me and my brother were little. It had taken several more years before he was persuaded to give up smoking in the car. Long, pre M4 journeys down to Cornwall, to holiday in my Great Auntie Vi's big green caravan, perched in her back garden, the sea in the distance, were always punctuated with smoking rows.

The journeys were also punctuated with ever increasing pleas of 'I don't feel very well', as mum scrabbled about for a carrier bag.

'Pull over Geoff, she's going to be sick,' mum would screech.

'I can't just pull over,' dad would shout.

I'm sure it's part of the reason why the smell of vomit makes me feel, well, sick. Not a great qualification for current circumstances, though at least here in hospital I just had to bundle the sheets up, not scrape it off before shoving it in the washing machine.

H and Pops both seemed pleased when dad woke up, but he didn't say very much, before falling asleep again.

'Are you sure dad's alright,' I asked mum, again.

'He's tired after driving, that's all,' said mum, 'he's not much company these days.'

By the time mum and dad had left with Pops, H was asleep. It was good knowing Pops was with them, she seemed almost excited about showing grandma and granddad around Charly's House and our phone call that night, taken on grandma's phone, was much calmer.

Lying on the now familiar narrow pull down bed, my mind refused to shut down. Their dad was due to visit the following day.

I couldn't sleep. Whether because I was on alert for H or because of the seemingly constant attention from nurses and doctors, which meant the room never felt private, I just couldn't switch off long enough to drop off.

I was concerned about how their dad would react to seeing H in such a state. He'd spent many long months in hospitals as a youngster. He had been born with club feet, to teenage parents, and had undergone a number of pioneering operations.

I knew he was confused about H's cancer and the treatment, that he believed his son was likely to die, even though Jamie had explained the protocols. Despite being a scientist himself, their dad didn't view the world like most of us.

That night, in trying to make sense of so many things, it was impossible not to re-examine the reasons why I had become a single parent.

I was 34 when we'd met, through a dating agency, before

internet dating and social media became a way of life. In theory I was matched with a number of 'suitable' men according to my background and interests. I think the old-fashioned approach had appealed to me, though it soon became apparent there was very little 'matching' going on. Just a lot of men looking for a woman.

I was never going to be compatible with a pet shop assistant from Basingstoke who didn't drive, or a man who drove a pink car and claimed to work for the MOD but couldn't talk about his job because he'd signed the Official Secrets Act. I had, too, as a student. Yup, had to sign in before I was allowed in to prison, where I spent my 21st, if you recall...

After a string of increasingly bizarre dates, I decided I was destined to be single, travel a lot and have cats. My now ex-husband had left a message on my answer machine and, because I felt guilty at not having replied sooner, I agreed to meet him for a drink, vowing it would be my last blind date for a very long time.

I should have gone home after first impressions. I wasn't attracted to him. But he seemed charming and intelligent. As he talked it felt like he'd never really talked to anyone like he did to me that first evening. It was endearing. I agreed to a second date.

He'd seemed genuine and I marvelled at all the books on his bookshelves which mirrored mine. He left bunches of long-stemmed red roses by my front door, bottles of Champagne.

Three months after meeting I discovered I was pregnant. In shock, not just at the failed condom but by my reproductive failings, I told him. He was so shocked he went out and bought a family pack of condoms. I should have known then that something was not quite right...

I told him he did not have to *stand by me*, but I could not have an abortion. No, I hadn't suddenly discovered religion. But to discover you are pregnant, at 34, having been told you will probably never have children, well – my biological grenade had just had the pin removed.

Twelve weeks into the pregnancy I had my hospital ceiling lights experience, the remains of our child were surgically removed under general anaesthetic. His response had been simply 'we can have more children'.

Just over six months after we met, on Christmas Eve and bended knee, he asked me to marry him. I said 'yes' and we married in the new Millennium, a year and a week after we'd met.

When I walked up the aisle, I was four months pregnant with H. The dressmakers were very understanding; it's hardly an original scenario.

Six weeks after the full white job, in a picture-perfect Dorset church, he confessed he had not been 'entirely honest' with me. By the time H was born I was frantically plastering over the cracks in our marriage as each new revelation emerged, while attempting to deal with his debts, which threatened to overwhelm everything, particularly when he lost his job.

I thought I'd got us back on track. I thought I could cope with his foibles and idiosyncrasies, even though by then we were in bedrooms as separate as the boxes he lived in inside his head. I felt we had both worked hard on moving forward and, one night, we cemented those feelings in time honoured fashion.

By the time I knew our marriage had no future I discovered I was pregnant with Pops. She was very definitely a child who wanted to be in this world! As friends joked, it only takes once...

Three weeks before Pops was born, I asked him to move out. Neither of us could have coped if we had stayed together, we would have destroyed each other. But it was me who had to make the decision and it is a decision I have never regretted.

I filed for divorce. It took two bloody and painful years to achieve, longer than the 22 months we were married. The Decree Absolute arrived on my door mat a couple of days before my fortieth birthday. He'd tried to take my home away from me. The courts said 'no'.

No straight jacket was unpacked during the obtaining of our divorce, though I must have frequently perused the catalogues. I made several quilts during that time.

It was always my belief, just because I messed up on marriage, that H and Pops should not suffer because of it. I felt by initiating proceedings when they were so young, we could create our own, 21st century family, which included their dad. It was hard work. It was painful and at times heart breaking. Yet it was why I had no angst about seeing him in Bristol. We were in regular contact and, particularly since we had moved to Devon, the relationship between all four of us had relaxed into comfortable territory. I'd worked hard to retain a friendship following divorce.

I still believe marriage is all too often a random experience undertaken by two people who are naïve. Yet I also have the pleasure of knowing many couples who are a living testament to the joys of finding your soul mate, spending the best of lifetimes revelling in each other's company. Yes, I admit it. I'm a romantic and a bloody divorce can't part me from my Piscean persona. Or maybe it was just the human condition, living in hope...

All I hoped for at that moment was H's health and Pops' presence. I had no way of knowing someone else was soon to be added on to my wish list, and it wasn't Father Christmas.

CHAPTER
TWENTY-SEVEN

THE SHEER VOLUME OF PEOPLE ENTERING AND LEAVING OUR LIVES FELT staggering. We said hello to Nic as he came to pick up Debbie, who we then had to say goodbye to. Within minutes Pops was missing her, but Nic had arrived with a tool box and fixed the gushing tap. It was a huge relief as there had still been no word from anyone regarding Charly's House.

Their dad called, delayed his visit to the following day, which was a relief as H was not doing great.

The blog summed up where we were at.

"H has had a challenging 36 hours. Spiking temperatures (lingo for up and down like crazy) so we didn't get much sleep last night. A CT scan revealed a fungal infection, for which he is now being treated. As well as anti-fungal medicine he is on various antibiotics, a saline drip (again), a night time feed, electrolytes as potassium levels are low and he is currently hooked up to a heart monitor. Tomorrow looks like another blood transfusion and maybe more platelets.

"We are going for every medicine and medical procedure possible in the first few weeks. If we get it over with now, maybe it'll get easier... It's all quite 'normal' apparently... We are still in isolation... While I am knackered, the men in white coats have yet to be called."

By then H and I had had the 'you-are-going-to-lose-all-your-hair' conversation. Clumps of it were already beginning to appear on his pillow. I was trying to get the hospital hairdresser to visit, to cut it short, but the words 'flu' and 'swine' had scared them off.

I had asked H if he'd like me to have all my hair cut off, too. It was fairly long, past my shoulders. He looked me in the eye for a second or two,

'Go on then Mum, yes. But how will you get it cut?' he said.

It was a good question. I'd have to ask around.

The blog offered up my feelings.

"Freely confess I'm not looking forward to H having a bald head. You think you are too tired to still be emotional, and then the smallest thing sets you off. Someone asked me today how I was getting on with the Christmas shopping. Then, of course, I thought 'OhMyGod... How will Father Christmas find us when I don't even know where we will be for Christmas? How will magic and stockings and chimneys and feeding reindeer enormous carrots and sprinkling fairy dust outside the front door and leaving sherry and mince pies on the fireplace be able to happen?

"Then you remember the old life, the life before leukaemia, the simplicity of our own private and personal little rituals which are now gone. Not forever, but they will never be the same again. Life will never be the same again, whatever the outcome. Once you have experienced a world which the majority knows nothing about, it separates you, it isolates you from other people. As we have yet to meet up with other parents in our situation, I do feel pretty alone in all this. If it wasn't for all the amazing support we are getting from friends and family I think I'd feel very lonely indeed...

"While I could really use a big masculine bear hug from someone who really knew me, I know so many people are really rooting for H. And mega news. My dad, after 55 years a smoker, has given up. Yup, at age 71 he's given up because of H's leukaemia. That's a small miracle in

itself. Even their dad has learnt to text... See how small things can change the world?

"H has just had two anti-sickness meds and some potassium through his feeding tube, so we must sleep. Who knows how tomorrow will play out? One step nearer to recovery. Another step away from the awful uncertainty, the downright fear of the unknown. Still, at least I know one thing – the hospital food will be another culinary foray into the unknown. Come on Jamie Oliver, we need you. OK, Nigella would be great, Hugh F-W a joy, Delia, Michel, Raymond, Nigel Slater. Where are you all hiding?"

I suspect I was beginning to fixate on food a little. H was now so emaciated he was being fed through a tube inserted down his left nostril, straight into his stomach. Bottles of yellow gunk – vanilla flavoured, which seemed utterly pointless if it was by-passing your taste buds and nasal passages – were being fed down the tube, at regular intervals, by yet another electronic pump. It was apparently a carefully formulated, nutritionally balanced substance which was used as a food replacement for patients too ill to eat.

Each time I gave H a drink I also had to add a powder called *Polycal,* formulated to get calories into sick people. It made any liquid so gloopy it couldn't be sucked through a straw. I had to write down everything H was eating and drinking, for the nutritionist and for the nurses.

The hospital food was lamentable. It was a double whammy for a foodie mum struggling to be able to nurture her children with lovingly prepared food. No kitchen, see.

H and Pops had been pushed and dragged around farmers markets and food fairs from a young age. Not just because I believed in decent, sustainable food but because I was lucky enough to have been a food writer for several years. I'd always been on the lookout for an exciting producer, someone hunting a new food sensation, anything unusual. Among my culinary highlights had been sipping peppermint tea on the banks of the Thames, in Bray, interviewing Michel Roux Senior, while Junior cooked in the kitchen. Raymond Blanc told me how he used to tie his mother to a chair so he could cook for her. Tim Burton-Race described how he'd fallen in love with his wife all over again, when they moved to France so he could spend a year cooking French. Rustie Lee was a scream, her Caribbean cookbook an education. I'd spoken to hot young Royal chefs, those who were the toast of the culinary scene, the innovators, movers and sprinklers. Obviously, I'd had to review restaurants, judge sausages, eat cake, eulogise about the latest cookery books. I'd loved every moment. It meant food had been a part of my children's growing up.

How far we had fallen. From long slow cooked shin of beef in red wine, calamari and garlic mayo, homemade ice creams, soups, fish pies and spaghetti Bolognese, homemade pizza. We were now on yellow gunk and piles of congealing brown stuff garnished with soggy veg and puddings in small plastic pots.

I had eaten little since we arrived in Bristol. People were beginning to comment on how much weight I was losing. I was noticing clothes feeling looser. But my elation was focused on getting through another day and spending time with Pops. Me and food would keep for another day, another chapter.

I must have slept at some point, only to be woken by a nurse checking H's vitals. I drifted off wondering how on earth I would be able to organise a Christmas for two children, who must surely have been at the top of Santa's list. Should I Google his address in Lapland, let him know where they were? Except I couldn't. No one knew where we'd be. Now there's a challenge for the man in red.

Perhaps I could entice him in with a luxury M&S mince pie, one of the ones stuffed with walnuts and brandy?

CHAPTER TWENTY-EIGHT

THE TIDE WAS TURNING, I COULD FEEL IT! H WAS STABLE AND POPS HAD had a good night, being with grandma a lovely distraction for her. And I was declared officially swine flu free. My concerns about dad were shunted out of my head by an astonishing piece of good luck.

I had started asking around if anyone knew a decent hairdresser. The ward's housekeeper, in daffodil yellow, had given me the number of hers, who happened to be close by, at the bottom of the gloriously named Christmas Steps. Incredibly, the salon owner had a cancellation for that morning.

Mum and dad were able to sit with H while Pops and I pottered off, the air crisp with adventure and December breath mist. While Pops was plied with chocolates and miniature mince pies, the deliciously camp crimper – OK, I don't like stereotypes but he was camper than Boy George and just as cheeky – listened. Give him credit, when faced with a slightly unhinged woman, he took it completely in his stride.

I launched into a clumsy monologue.

'My son is in hospital. He's got cancer and he's going to lose all his hair and so I asked him if he wanted me to have all mine cut off and he said yes, so I was wondering if, err, you could cut all my hair off. Please.'

He stood behind me, the scissors in his left hand balanced on his hip as he walked around me, lifting strands, running his fingers through my hair which had, actually received attention a few months previously.

'No,' he said, 'I won't cut all your hair off.'

'But I promised my son' I said. 'He's going to lose all his and I said I would...'

'It's OK, I'll cut it short,' he said, cutting me off (excuse the pun!) 'But very short won't suit you. I'll give you some shape here' and he gestured with both hands, 'and here. Then we'll lift this at the side ... with some layering here and, yes, that's going to look great.'

By the time Pops was almost sick from chocolate, and I'd been relieved of a week's worth of grocery money, we were walking away on a cloud of hairspray and *product*. It was the best cut I'd had in years. If ever. Was it awful to feel so thrilled I'd had such a decent haircut, when the only reason for it was my son's cancer-induced hair loss?

Back in Room 4 Pops insisted on taking some pictures of my new almost elfin haircut, a cut which harked back to my early twenties when my skin had been brighter and my twinkle shinier. A few frames along and there were pictures of H with a number two, his scalp showing in patches.

The hospital hairdresser had not only failed to show up, she hadn't even answered any phone calls. When the ward couldn't locate any clippers one of the youngest nurses had, on her day off, gone into Bristol and bought some. When I jelly wobbled at having to shave my son's hair, which had to be snipped away first because it was so long, other Very Young nurse had stepped into the breach.

H's transformation was almost complete. No makeup department needed to transform him into an extra on *The Boy in the Striped Pyjamas.* Not once did H complain. He smiled throughout and grinned at the camera for his 'close up'.

I'd thought I was getting the hang of the blog, writing it in the dark perched on the side of the pull-down bed.

"Have just written what I thought was around 700 funny words on H's current hair status, only to find I have pressed some invisible delete button. I just don't believe it – bet everyone reading this does though. Will attempt to rewrite from memory later today as now so knackered am bound to keep pressing the invisible delete key...

"Oh yes, and H's swine flu has mutated. We truly are at the cutting edge of the most fashionable virus on earth. Still, at least it means we remain on top of the 'you couldn't make it up' league tables.

Love to all, I will catch up with you all in time,

Crazy Blood Mum xxx"

CHAPTER TWENTY-NINE

I WAS BEGINNING TO FEEL LIKE A HOTEL DOORMAN IN CHARGE OF A FINE set of polished revolving doors, without the brass buttons and perky hat.

As mum and dad left, their dad was expected, along with my primary school friend Lizzie. We had known each other since the age of six.

We tried to meet up when we could as adults, but the gaps increased between visits, yet it would take moments for us to key back into each other's lives and before long we'd be jabbering away as if over our garden fences.

I still marvelled at our enduring friendship. Lizzie left school at sixteen and went to work in a bank. I left school at eighteen, ploughed my A levels and had a year off, working in a printing factory while doing retakes at night school, before heading to West Yorkshire as a student.

By the time I'd graduated, toiled in France for six months and was on my first paper as a cub reporter, Lizzie was married and a nurse. She had suitcases and a spare room, I had backpacks. Lizzie married her second husband before I even contemplated my first. Lizzie had a teenage step daughter and I had H and Pops. Lizzie was petite, neat and glamorous; I'm large, wild and rarely coordinated.

One of the emergency emails I'd sent, on that wet and wild night three weeks ago, had been to Lizzie. She had been due to come and stay with us and I'd had to cancel. And here's friendship for you! She juggled her life and came to see us anyway, in Bristol, bearing pyjamas for H and Pops, sanity for me.

Of course we hugged. And of course we cried. She arrived late on Friday night, after a full day at work and after a catch up she whisked Pops off to Charly's House so they could both unwind and get some sleep. And she promised to take up the swine flu gauntlet and spend the following night with H in Room 4, so I could have a night with Pops. She was the only person in the world I would have allowed to do it. She was a nurse; she knew her stuff and H was happy about it. Pops was ecstatic.

It was a relief she had arrived safely after a long drive. I knew H was very tired. Their dad had come to see them both, arriving with chocolate from great grandma, the best Green and Blacks had to offer.

Becky had also come to visit, bringing home made cakes and eggs from the chickens who were, by all accounts thriving, their battery days well behind them. Korma was particularly happy, reported Becky, much to our amusement. She also brought news about the cats. While Julie was still feeding them before and after the school run, other grandma had been persuaded to have Oscar, where he would have huge gardens to mouse in and be company for other granddad indoors. Ruby was nesting in with Becky's brood. The relief was immense, though I was a bit concerned for Oscar. He didn't travel well.

It was just H and I, ten o'clock vitals were completed without drama and it felt as if we could both breathe. It was early days with the vile black spores but there was no deterioration. I attended to the night time feed. As each day passed, I was able to do more administering to H. The nurses actively encouraged it. No, you're OK, I won't be unleashing myself into the world of nursing anytime soon, but he was my child and there was nothing I wouldn't have done for him. Or for my daughter. Damn, should have signed up for an NVQ or some such. There's nothing like a good bit of solid learning to keep you on your toes. How to combat cancer with half a cucumber?

Reflecting on my funky new hair cut in the en suite mirror led to another revelation of increasingly staggering proportions. Or rather, decreasing proportions. Even I could see how much weight I was losing. Was it bad to feel good about it? Rather than reflecting on my weight, a dangerous obsession, I sat with H and read to him. As he fell asleep, I stroked his scalp, which was beginning to resemble a moth-eaten scrubbing brush. Not a good look.

At last, a moment of calmness, possibly the first in three weeks. Earlier in the day I had received a phone call, one I hadn't dared to hope was the one call I so desperately needed.

My caring friend Jude, down in Devon, the friend I had begged to come and help us because she was a professional carer, had come up with an idea. Well, a person. Jude met Magda in a children's home. It's OK, they were both staff and fully CRB checked, referenced up to the hilt.

By a rather uncanny string of coincidences Magda was between contracts from the beginning of January, and her personal life could suddenly dovetail in with our requirements. Jude was convinced she could talk to Magda and suggest we met up to discuss the possibility of her becoming Pops' carer, five days a week. A sleep-in carer.

The plan was for Jude to speak to Magda and see if she would consider the possibility. Jude would then drive Magda to Bristol to meet us. Then it was up to me to persuade her it could work. She would be a 'nanny', in somewhat intense conditions. It was a big ask. I could only wait and keep my fingers crossed.

If Magda said 'yes', I had a way forward. And she was known by a friend of mine, whose judgement I trusted implicitly. All I had to figure was how I would pay her. At least I now had cheque books in Bristol, thanks to Becky and Julie. But you can't write cheques if there's nothing to back them up. Yes, I know someone should have told the bankers, but I like to think I take a more honest approach to life.

Although I did once write a cheque to buy an Interrail ticket, which gave me access to Europe by rail for a month, knowing there wasn't quite enough to cover it before I went. By God it was worth the letters afterwards. Paid it all off with the late summer job and it meant I got to see my still favourite place in the world – the Djemaa-el-Fna in Marrakesh, Morocco - and The Alhambra Palace in Grenada, Spain. It had been a risk, but I never regretted that particular indiscretion.

I had to trust Magda was another risk worth taking – if she agreed. Then all I had to do was write a job description.

And print a few thousand pounds to pay her.

Then I got another phone call. Other grandma had lasted less than 12 hours with Oscar Wilde. She couldn't cope with his meowing, so had driven the poor little bugger back to ours. He was now a cat without a lap. Why on earth had I agreed to let other grandma take him? She made my mum look like a very responsible adult ...

CHAPTER THIRTY

IT WAS GREAT TO SPEND TIME WITH LIZZIE ON SATURDAY, THE FOUR OF US holed up in Room 4, catching up. H fancied a tomato, so Pops and I went shopping. I bought a punnet of beautiful, totally out of season baby plum ones in, yes, our closest food hall. He nibbled one, the rest sat on the window sill.

His taste buds were reacting to the chemo drugs. He wanted sour foods. I say 'foods', he wasn't really eating but I tried to find things which might appeal to his jaded palate. Lemon sherbets and lemonade made with real lemons were a hit, though I was now worrying about his teeth. Nutritionally he was still on yellow gunk three times a day. At least the sickness and diarrhoea had abated, though he had such a red bum I was worried about it becoming infected.

It seemed minor in the scheme of things, a sore bum. But an infected scratch can kill and his emaciated body was already fighting cancer, mutated swine flu and an evil fungus which probably wasn't black at all. He was also due to start taking Relenza because doctors wanted to try and clear up the swine flu more quickly.

Although on-going lab tests showed H's swine flu had

mutated, I didn't know into what. It's not as if he'd turned into a piglet! It only took a small change in the virus DNA for a mutation, but just two mutations had the power to change the course of a pandemic. I'd been doing some homework.

Headlines proclaimed scientists feared a significant mutation of the H1N1 virus could follow a pattern seen in previous flu outbreaks; a mild version spread around the world, then evolved into a more virulent, deadlier second wave. Maybe one day someone would write a paper on H's mutation. Or, most likely, it was an insignificant change and would fade into a line in his medical records.

I have avoided the word *stoic,* but he was. Despite everything H even laughed when I joked it was just like when he was a baby, me cleaning his bum.

'Oh Mum,' he said, 'I'm not going back into nappies!'

Lizzie was wonderful. There were no dramas during the night and it meant Pops and I were able to stay together in Charly's House. I was upset at how stark her bedroom looked. But of course it was; all she had were a pile of inadequate clothes, Leemy, some comics and a book, plus a pink fleecy blanket Hayley had given her. And some bunting, with letters spelling out POPS, made for her by The Evening Stars, which we draped as we couldn't hang them anywhere. Her toothbrush and a tube of toothpaste lay on the side of the sink in the empty en suite bathroom of her top floor bedroom, the brown towels and two single beds as neutral as everything else in the house. I felt she was invisible, like a mouse living in a hole behind the skirting board.

'We need to make this into your bedroom, Pops. Let's go shopping,' I said, trying to find reasons to be cheerful.

'I just want to be with you and H,' she wailed.

All I could say as I hugged her was 'I know love, I know. And tomorrow you will be.'

'Oh yes, I will be,' and she perked right up.

When Pops finally fell asleep I got out of the other single bed in her room and went down a flight of stairs to the living room. It was the first time I had sat on a sofa in three weeks. I had to open the sash window of the living room as wide as it would go, the room was so hot. But I was worried about turning the boiler off in case it wouldn't go back on again.

The view out of the window was stunning. Bristol blazed in all its twinkling night time glory. I could see the hotel where Pops had slept. I could see much of the panoramic breadth of this city of hills. I could breathe in the tranquillity which can only be found in the late night of an early morning. Night time is my time and dark brings out magic. Though my heart lay in the rocks of Dartmoor, its secret forests and the salty skylines of my soul, I was now drinking in the beauty of this new-to-me city. Maybe we could become friends? If we were to survive this experience. I'd have to get to know it; there is always salvation in exploration.

Dragging myself away from the window, I knew I needed sleep while I could get it.

Waking up in a bed next to my daughter was sheer joy, but spurred our return to H.

Lizzie had to leave on the Sunday afternoon and my friend Sandra – yes, stitcher Sandra - was coming on Monday evening after work. In a miraculous twist of fate Sandra found herself between contracts, able to commit to helping us for the next two weeks.

The relief was immense, it bought us time. If Magda could only say yes...

Testing out the hospital's promise to be flexible, I had asked if Pops could stay in Room 4 on Sunday night. 'They' consented. Becky had brought up, at my request, our sleeping bags and camping mats, so we were all set. (No child-size mattresses in a paediatric oncology ward?) Sleeping on the floor was a small price to pay for having both my children in the same room overnight.

Apart from waving Lizzie off, Sunday heralded two significant phone calls.

The first was from Jude. Magda had agreed to meet me in Bristol, to talk about the possibility of becoming a paid carer for Pops five days a week. We were due to meet ten days before Christmas. I was elated.

The second call I made, to my brother.

I was becoming increasingly concerned about our father. For some time I had been aware his behaviour was best described as 'erratic'. I say behaviour, I meant mostly our interactions over the phone. We were not a close family. My mum is not a matriarchal character.

Mum had stepped up, looked after H and Pops when I'd had the chance for an adventure or two. Thanks to her I'd made it to Amsterdam, Santiago de Compostela in Spain and fitted in a barmy coach trip to a clutch of German Christmas Markets. I had been very grateful for those snatched opportunities; it kept the dust off my passport.

During my growing up years dad, a quantity surveyor, had renovated our homes as a hobby, and immersed himself in local politics at both town and county level. I grew up in beautifully decorated homes with tidy gardens, yet spent very little time with my dad. I left home just before I turned nineteen.

We were, however, very alike, me and my dad. At times fiery with each other – which mum hated – but our outlooks were similar and we were both aspiring writers and frustrated thespians.

I knew my dad wasn't right. Seeing him a couple of days earlier confirmed my feelings. We'd had some odd phone calls in recent months, where he'd go off at a tangent or change the subject for no reason. Each time I tried to speak to mum her response was 'he's fine'. I had persisted and mum admitted he'd had some memory tests via the GP, which hadn't flagged up any particular concerns. She did, however, regularly complain about him moving things and then not remembering where he'd put them. Or parking the car and then not being able to find it.

My alarm bells were ringing. I rang my brother, hoping to have a chat about what he thought.

'Hello Neil, it's me,' I said, the mobile bleeping unhelpfully. 'How are you doing?'

'I'm fine. How's H?' I knew he was upset about H. We lived 160 odd miles apart and didn't see each other very often, but he got on well with his niece and nephew. He was also their Godfather.

We had a bit of a chat, then I launched.

'Neil, we need to talk about Dad,' I said.

'There's nothing to talk about,' he said.

The phone call didn't last much longer. Christmas was mentioned. And that, was that.

The real sadness was knowing there was nothing I could do for my dad.

I was marooned in Bristol and I had no choice but to be a mother, not a daughter.

CHAPTER
THIRTY-ONE

THE ATMOSPHERE IN ROOM 4 WAS 'HOLIDAY'. AFTER RELUCTANTLY SAYING goodbye to Lizzie, Pops and I chose a pile of DVDs from the Ward 34 'library'. In reality it was H and Pops discussing what might be on the shelves and me, who was now 'allowed' out of the room because of my newly acquired 'swine flu-free status', popping out to have a rootle.

We 'bedded in' for the evening. Pops lay next to H on his bed, me encased in blankets and sleeping bags balanced on the turquoise chair, legs stretched across the bottom of the bed. We set up the TV, its extended wire stretched across the ceiling, which also made a handy washing line. Very 'health and safety'.

We revisited 'The Secret Garden', watched 'The Bee Movie' and discussed the ethics of 'stealing' honey from our stripy friends, then became immersed in the world of Wallace and Gromit – Aardman Animations continue to be a huge supporter of Bristol Children's Hospital.

H remained stable. He was ministered to regularly and we three enjoyed a glorious Sunday, punctuated by microwave popcorn, ready meals from our closest food hall and, for H, a steady stream of lemon sherbets interspersed with yellow gunk.

Did I imagine the blood transfusion, for dramatic effect, as things seemed so drama free?

It was our calmest night in three weeks. All of us managed some sleep and I was so grateful to the nursing staff who never once made me feel in the way with my Bedouin-style encampment, on the floor at the bottom of H's bed.

Sunday set the tone for the following week.

Sandra arrived on Monday evening, fresh from work and the train journey. Pops had known Sandra since she was a new born and was excited she was coming. I was confident the next two weeks would be able to offer Pops some stability. My feelings towards my sewing buddy, and her other half Alan, had often gone beyond words.

We met after putting our names on a list at a textile exhibition in Reading, declaring our interest in joining a new patchwork group. Sandra spotted we both lived in the same road and knocked on my door. I opened it to a petite blonde and we burbled our way into friendship.

When their dad and I separated, Sandra gave unconditional support. Three weeks after Pops was born my back went. I ended up on crutches, at times only able to crawl on my hands and knees. It meant I couldn't carry baby Pops up, or down, the stairs. Sandra arrived each morning on her way to work and carried her down for me. Each bedtime she came over and carried Pops back up again. Thank goodness we had a downstairs bathroom.

With Sandra in Bristol life became easier. Spotting the growing mountain of over flowing re-useable bags in the corner of the room, which now included Christmas shopping, she took on the mission of getting it all to Charly's House. Each day Sherpa Sandra filled her rucksack and carried bags, with Pops' help, up the steepest of hills. It was staggering how much 'stuff' had ended up in the room. It was, in so many ways, the embodiment of the support and generosity from so many, as if people were trying to create a sticking plaster of kindness made of 'stuff'.

I had failed to keep up with it all and lost track of where it all came from. My mind had been so focused on H and Pops any detail that was not essential to getting H well, and keeping Pops with us, got lost.

A new sense of order was emerging in our hospital life and each day that week H made progress. On Wednesday I had a meeting with CLIC social worker, Lin. There was no grant towards a carer for Pops, but Lin's knowledge and practical suggestions were invaluable.

Throughout the week Jamie was a regular presence, his leukaemia knowledge offered incredible reassurance and there was nothing I couldn't ask him. He faultlessly trod the line between professionalism, and friendship.

Jamie was part funded by CLIC Sargent; Lin was wholly funded by them. So many people we had never met – people who sponsored walks, shaved their heads, ran marathons – were willing us on. Those thoughts were empowering.

Their dad came to visit on Thursday, bringing several original Dr Who DVDs, which kept H entertained for hours on end. I found the familiarity of Tom Baker's voice oddly reassuring, though what I really wanted was a visit from David Tennant, or a hug from John Barrowman, AKA Captain Jack. *'Mum, you do know he's gay, don't you?'* chorused H and Pops. And?

Their dad was always uncomfortable in a new environment. He had very little to say to his son or daughter. I was too tired to keep a conversation going, he quietly blended into our alien landscape, his left leg tapping against the chair leg. I think his presence was enough, particularly for H. They had a real connection with the whole Dr Who phenomenon.

H's hair loss was difficult to witness, but their dad couldn't talk about any of it, just as he never talked about anything personal. He stayed for a couple of hours, did his usual 'got to go now', stood up and left. H and Pops were by then used to their dad's mannerisms, it wasn't odd for them.

On Friday Sandra had to return to Reading for a work commitment. Pops went with her, on the train. I hoped the adventure would be a break for Pops, give her some relief from the in-your-face existence she had been forced to confront each day.

It meant H and I had a whole weekend to ourselves. It meant H could really get some rest. Visitors are great but they heap pressure on to hospital living. At times Room 4 felt like a heated waiting room at Victoria Station.

Saturday morning sunshine – one of those cold, bright days just like the day of diagnoses four weeks ago – lured me out of Room 4. The nurses promised me H would be fine for an hour or two. I'd heard about a fabric shop the other side of the city centre and, promising to bring something back for H, I headed out. It was so good to walk, briskly, the excitement of a new project on the horizon.

I love the book title 'Chicken Soup for the Soul'. Fabric shops are my 'chicken soup' – Jewish chicken soup, of course my dear. It was Hanukkah. *The Festival of Lights*. I don't know why I have always enjoyed the idea of such a festival, Diwali as well. Maybe we are all connected to this world by ancient rituals we know little of. Or maybe I just approach fabric shops with a sense of reverence and awe.

H was excited when I arrived back in Room 4, face cold from the frosty air, two carrier bags of goodies. For him I bought Binca – pre-holed stiff fabric great for embroidery stitches you can turn into bookmarks– along with some bright embroidery threads and large eyed needles.

For myself I bought calico and felt, lots of sequins, beads and organic-coloured cottons, fine eyed beading needles. A vague idea was forming, after seeing a festive folk-art tree in a sewing magazine. One month in and I was sewing star-shaped sequins onto fabric.

The only thing which pricked our little bubble that weekend was Pops. She was struggling.

Sandra took her to see friends in Reading. I had felt a trip to Cathy's, the chance to play with their four children in their familiar family home, would be calming. Cathy – my psychologist friend Dr Leather – described her as a 'lost child'.

Each phone call we had with Pops was tear-filled. I couldn't wait for her to come back to hospital.

CHAPTER THIRTY-TWO

The return of Pops was a boost. H had developed an allergy to the Relenza, leaving him with a nasty rash. Despite a quiet weekend he was exhausted. I thought he'd been given steroids at some point, to help with the rash. It was hard to tell if the raised temperature was another infection or his body's response to so many chemicals. Or the leukaemia.

The blog read;

"We are still in isolation, though Pops is now also free of swine flu... H is recovering from the nasty rash caused by the Relenza and they will re-test (him) again soon.

"This week H is likely to be having his second bone marrow sample taken under a general, so the docs can assess treatment so far and see where we go from here. Learning curve still immense. H has now lost nearly all his hair (it's darn powerful that chemo!) but we have put up plenty of Christmas decs ... so the future is currently looking pretty and sparkly.

"...Typing in the dark is not ideal – it's a bit like reporting from the frontline... guess I am really, the frontline against Crazy Blood."

I was nervous about meeting Magda the following day. I could only hope we got on, that she decided to get involved and take the job. Crikey, if she did, I'd suddenly become a boss.

It was so good to spend time with Pops. The feeling hardened my resolve to make sure things worked with Magda. She HAD to say yes. There was, at that point, absolutely no alternative. I knew I could find a way of sorting the money. I did some sums. Lizzie had started the ball rolling; she had paid £500 into my bank account. I was bowled over.

'Look Sharon, you have to accept it,' she said, 'it's just money and you need it.'

I spoke to Jude. She would drive to Bristol the following afternoon, with Magda. They would come up to Room 4, meet H and Pops. Then we would go and get a coffee somewhere so I could interview Magda.

Monday night I managed little sleep, attempting to write a job description and figure out what I could afford to pay Magda, plus a bit, in a bid get her on board.

The phone rang. It was Cathy, Dr Leather.

'Sharon, we want to give you some money. Mark and I feel you need this, it's a gift. We were thinking of giving you money at Christmas, for a holiday or something, anyway.'

I was stunned, and told I was not allowed to argue. Cathy and Mark were giving me £2,000. We agreed it was best to use it to pay Magda.

It meant I could meet Magda later in the day with confidence. I knew I could pay her for at least two months, the rest I would sort, somehow.

It was great to see Jude, just a couple of hours later. Hugs and held back tears over, it was time to contemplate the serious looking young woman who was talking to H and Pops.

I was impressed her priority was to talk to them.

'You must be Pops' said Magda, smiling. 'Which means you must be H,' she said, walking to the bed.

'Are you Jude's friend?' said H, 'Mum's told us about you. Are you going to come and live in Bristol with us?'

I cringed a bit. Don't pre-empt, don't scare her off...

Neat and serious summed up what I saw. She spoke with a pronounced Polish accent, her grammar was perfect and her vocabulary wide, if the colloquialisms peppering conversation were anything to go by.

I had to make decisions. Did I like her because I felt I had to, because I had no choice? Or were my instincts genuine?

By the time we had drunk coffee in The Wild Wood, a café at the front of the hospital, I felt I had asked as many questions as I possibly could. Jude was a huge support and, with her knowledge of the care industry, we agreed a deal which I felt appealed to Magda.

'I think it is better for me to sleep over Sunday night,' said Magda. 'I think it will be easier for you to find help from friends on Friday and Saturday night.'

I liked her common sense attitude. She was bang on.

I offered to take her to Charly's House, on the proviso she understood by the time she came back to Bristol our accommodation was most likely to be CLIC House, which had an entirely different set up.

We didn't talk 'ifs'. It was definitely 'whens'.

At Charly's House I offered wine, Magda opted for coffee. She approved of my coffee pot, which Julie had brought up from Devon. I downed a large red, mentally toasting Hayley. It wasn't that I felt like celebrating, but Magda accepting the job was such a huge relief. Massive!

Magda would arrive in Bristol in January, and I would pay her to care for Pops from each Sunday night through to Friday morning. Between us we would juggle daytimes and I promised Magda plenty of free time whenever possible. At some point, if H was well enough and Magda chose to, maybe she could sleep in the hospital occasionally?

'Yes, but of course, that will be fine,' she said.

I would have to continue putting together a weekend diary, of people who could come and look after Pops.

In a flurry of emotional hugs – well, you wouldn't expect my hugs not to be emotional, would you? – Magda and Jude set off into the dark night.

I walked back to the hospital, going down Leg Wobble Hill, so Sandra and Pops could come back to Charly's House for the night. It was cold. The sky was ink black, despite all the light pollution. It felt good to walk, to be out, to be on my own. Events were happening so fast it was almost as if my head simply couldn't keep up. Life was surreal. Small moments of head space were to be grasped whenever possible.

Maybe I was light headed from a second swift large red. I felt the embodiment of a surrealist painting; a Salvador Dali with body parts floating in the sky, out of proportion feet, no arms, my head filled with multiple spheres, drawers with knobs emerging from my legs, spikes, sticks, flames everywhere. Or maybe I was just losing it – the perfect model for a painting, if an artist could see what was going on inside my head.

As I neared the hospital one thought occurred. I had agreed to employ Magda, but I hadn't asked H and Pops what they thought of her. What if they didn't like her? Had I really thought this one through? Was there a choice?

Despite me refusing to accept the idea of Pops going into temporary foster care, CLIC Lin had made some inquiries. Even if it had been an avenue I'd consented to explore, it would have met a dead end. Lin discovered Bristol Social Services would not assist in a placement because we didn't live in Bristol. Devon County Council had also refused to discuss the scenario because, they said, we no longer lived in Devon. So where ...?

Outside in. Once more we were on the outside, looking in. We had fallen between the cracks in files on desks. We were at the bottom of a heap of papers, edited out of reality, an unsolvable problem. Cue chorus of *'How do you solve a problem like Maria?'*. Substitute *Sharon...* Not quite the same ring to it, but we were clearly a problem for the authorities so, best way to deal with us – pass the buck. Problem sorted.

When I got back to Room 4, slightly puffed as I was using the stairs rather than the lift, to get some exercise, I got three expectant looks.

'Well, how did you get on?' said Sandra.

'Did you like her,' I said, 'did you like Magda?'

H said 'yes' straight away.

Pops said she thought she did.

'Will she be a carer for me mummy?' she said.

'That's the general plan,' I said. 'She's due to start after New Year.'

'OK,' said Pops. And that was that.

Nothing in writing, no contract; simply a verbal agreement, a start date and a hug. It seemed my management style was based on the *'wing and a prayer'* model.

The phone rang. It was mum. We were speaking most days, it meant she felt in our loop.

'I've got some news for you, Sharon. At last, some good news. Well, I've got a cheque for £2,000 for you, from a couple at church. Isn't that great!'

How was it possible in one day – just one day – an entire thought process had become a realisable plan? It was extraordinary.

'Oh mum, that's fantastic,' I said, my throat catching.

I told her about Magda.

'That's brilliant news Sharon! Brilliant. How's H?'

Pops and Sandra left for the night. I felt numb with relief.

Exhausted. I looked around Room 4. It did look very Christmassy. Pops and I had found the new pound shop in town.

I slept, knowing I could impart good news to the meeting I was due to attend the following afternoon with several of the senior management team, including Doctor John and Jamie. Despite my own practical difficulties, I didn't believe the management to be obstructive, merely caught between the proverbial rock and hard place. Maybe our situation was unique.

Tomorrow I could tell them about Magda. Tomorrow I hoped to get a clearer idea of exactly where we were at in H's treatment plan. Tomorrow would surely bring us one day closer to going home.

CHAPTER THIRTY-THREE

THE MEETING WENT WELL. THE PLAN WAS TO GET H OUT OF HOSPITAL IN time for Christmas. It was great news because it meant all his blood counts were going in the right direction. He was neutropenic, which meant he had no immune system. But providing all components of his blood continued to recover, he would be allowed out of hospital for a few days.

If he remained stable, he could leave hospital for an hour or two. It was a revelation. I hoped I could find his shoes. We could show him Charly's House. I was warned, however, not to allow anyone else in a lift with us. One sneeze could cause immeasurable damage to such a compromised, immature immune system.

The weather got colder. Snow was forecast. For two days we had a stream of visitors.

Mum and dad arrived on Thursday. H was allowed out of hospital and mum cooked a roast chicken dinner at Charly's House. It felt like a celebration. I thought my dad looked tired. We never had the chance for a proper conversation. I was scared to ask if he'd done the driving.

Mum had made H and Pops a Christmas stocking each. I was

very touched. I sewed on some loops and buttons so we could hang them up.

At the weekend H's best friend, Isabella, came with her family, the 'Manaton Mob'. Mum Julie knew the route to Bristol Children's Hospital pretty well by then. Dad Richard – Techy Husband of laptop procurement scenario – braved the city centre to get us a dongle. With no internet connection in Charly's House, it was essential. They brought with them two huge Christmas stockings made at school, one each for H and Pops. H's was a patchwork of jewel colours, filled with gifts from all his class mates. Of course I cried.

His class mates and teachers had been incredibly supportive since we arrived in Bristol. There had been an avalanche of goodwill, huge hand-made cards and gifts. The teachers had not only sent a box of presents for me, but they donated all the money they would have spent on a Secret Santa. Julie handed me an envelope stuffed with cash. Of course I cried.

I had managed to buy some little bells for H's Year at school, and attached a named gift tag to each one, signed from the three of us. It felt like such a tiny gesture, but I was chuffed to be able to send something back.

As if whisked in by a tornado worthy of the Land of Oz, other grandma appeared. Despite her unpredictability she brought a touch of magic to proceedings; inner child and all that. She had carried with her plenty of Christmas surprises for their stockings.

It was great to see her with her grandchildren. I think she hid her shock at H's appearance very well. She also looked tired. I knew it was tough going with hubby. He was ill, but she was her usual vague self. I had no clue what the problem was. I'm not sure she really knew either.

It began to feel as if my children would have a Christmas after all. Pops and I had hung decorations all over Charly's House, strung up the cards arriving daily. I tried not to think about how much stuff we were accumulating. How on earth would I get it all to CLIC House? Don't think, just get on with it, said inner-voice-of-mildly-rising panic.

What mattered was their excitement. For me the thought all three of us could be together for a few days was the biggest gift of all.

In what turned out to be our last night in hospital before Christmas, H tested negative for swine flu. He'd been fighting it for almost seven weeks and now it was gone. Celebrations were stacking up faster than a box of chocolates could empty.

It was feeling like Christmas. The house looked festive, the fridge freezer was filling with food, the boiler was keeping a small sub-station busy and the under-stair cupboard was stuffed with presents. I'd have to put my mind to a tree.

The only thing that gave the game away was a double cupboard in the kitchen. Right across its three shelves was an array of drugs including antibiotics, anti-fungals, anti-sickness, syringes, creams, yellow gunk, tiny bottles of water to flush out H's wiggly, between meds, and a host of medical paraphernalia which could have stocked a small branch of Boots.

It freaked me out because I was about to become totally responsible for H's medical welfare in the coming few days. Sandra, ever practical, made a chart for me, with tick boxes, so I could ensure I'd done everything properly. It gave me even more respect for our nurses. How did they keep it all in their heads?

Sandra escaped Bristol before the snow arrived, just in time to catch the four inches which settled in Reading.

Had I known how disruptive the worst weather to hit Bristol in living memory was going to become, I would have cried.

CHAPTER THIRTY-FOUR

I couldn't believe my eyes. In the charity shop window, on the way to the Co-op behind Charly's House, stood an artificial Christmas tree. Almost up to my bust, it was the perfect height for the corner of our borrowed living room. It had seen better days, but when I looked more closely it had a vintage feel, the baubles and bows held on by grubby bits of old pipe cleaner.

The faded plastic green of the obviously artificial branches somehow added to its charm. Even better it was reduced to just £3. I saw the invisible Paddington-esque 'Please Look After This Tree' label, and knew it had to come 'home' with me.

Slight problem: the shop was closed.

Still, if I was really clever about this, I could nip back at opening time the following morning and snap it up. I couldn't believe it was still there, so glorious was it in its tackiness. But most importantly it meant I could give my children a tree at Christmas.

The irony wasn't lost on me. I am probably the most ardent anti artificial Christmas tree person in the entire world. I can't bear them. When they became really trendy in the 1970's my

Mum had bought one – in John Lewis (!). It had been white and sparkly and such models are still revered today... I'd hated it.

Real Christmas trees appeal to my pagan leanings. You bring greenery into the house to remind yourself, despite being deep in winter, spring is coming. The smell of spruce and pine and the dropping of needles is as much a part of a winter celebration as vases of fresh daffodils speak spring, June strawberries herald glorious summer days and conkers and pumpkins jump up and down proclaiming autumn.

So what are we doing in these consumer crazed, earth-destroying days? Manufacturing a load of plastic artificial trees which insulate lofts and cellars, come in and out of fashion as fast as sell by dates on Avocados, and ultimately end up in landfill.

All these thoughts, as I stood on the icy pavement outside the Hospice charity shop: I want that Christmas tree. I wish I could buy it now. What on earth am I thinking?

I'm thinking I need to make our Christmas as normal as possible. I have no idea where we'll actually be. In hospital or in Charly's House. We're miles away from home and all the familiar little and large decorations collected over so many years – before and after children – are sitting in bits of tissue paper and old Christmas wrapping paper in boxes in my loft. All those 'First Christmas' artefacts, crude school-made decorations one can never get rid of, Christmas stockings with memories laced into every stitch are inaccessible. I am creating Christmas from scratch because I want some 'normal' for my children. I am trying to create normal in a world where normal does not exist. I am on the outside looking in.

At home, in our small courtyard garden, I have a spindly yet beautiful Christmas tree which I bought for H's second Christmas. Each year since it has come into our home, to be decorated. Each year it stands proudly. Each year I wonder if it will make it to the next and each year it sprouts just enough more needles and branches for its survival as our next Christmas tree.

The tree has become an object of ridicule for some of our friends. But increasingly that tree, grown as tall as I am when we left Devon last month, is becoming revered by others. That tree is earning its own respect and it puts a smile on my face just thinking about it. It's green in every sense, and had earned its place in our family history.

If I don't move my butt, move away from the charity shop window, my feet will freeze to the pavement and I will fail in today's mission. Move on from the memories lady. There will be precious little food in our cupboards over Christmas if I don't walk away. I turn my attention to the task in hand; my Dickensian Christmas window drooling moment over. I steal myself to take on the snow and ice carpeting the entire pavement, cross the slippery slush of the road towards the back-street Co-op – so familiar I could almost be back at home – and attempt to focus on what I need to buy. Every single food opportunity must be covered so whatever H wants to eat while he may, or may not be out of hospital, is catered for.

I also have to try and work out just what I am able to carry. Walking is tricky now it has snowed and I am terrified – absolutely terrified – of falling over and breaking an arm or a leg. Having already had two painful falls I have a number of very purple bruises and a sore back. Breathe, says Inner Goddess, who is feeling a tad chilly by this point. And don't forget the Brussels sprouts, she added. Oh go on then, a bottle of sherry too. Dad will appreciate that. Just remember you have to carry it all...

To say I had felt like an Antarctic explorer who'd lost his dogs wasn't far off the mark by the time I got back to Charly's House. Under normal conditions it would take less than ten minutes. But the trek back had taken more than half an hour. The muscles in both arms were screaming for mercy from laden bags, my left shoulder burned like hell and my feet were wet and frozen through. But I was smiling my head off as I let myself in through the front door. The silent house beckoned. I emptied five bags of food and drink into the fridge and into the cupboards.

OK, so I know it sounds pretty dull sharing that with you but the sense of achievement in such a simple task was enormous. So what, she's done a bit of shopping. But it meant we should have plenty to get us through if we were lucky enough to escape hospital – and it meant I had enough to feed other people too.

The sense of satisfaction was, however, short lived. Now I had to get back to the hospital. I didn't even bother with a cuppa, simply donned boots and coat and gloves and set off in the dying light of a snowy, low sunned December day, back to Ward 34.

Please don't let me fall over, went today's mantra, as I moved slower than a ninety-year-old, holding on to bushes, brick walls and iron railings as I went. Somehow, I had to get down that steep hill without slithering my way to the Bristol Royal Infirmary A&E department, which happened to be at the bottom.

Hold on Goddess, here we go!

It was the closest I'd ever got to extreme sports.

CHAPTER THIRTY-FIVE

A TAXI DROPPED THE THREE OF US IN THE UNLOADING BAY OF THE hospital, right opposite the sliding doors. It was Christmas Eve morning and the hospital was busy.

Everyone milling seemed to have a purpose speeded up by tinsel tied to aprons, daft Christmas earrings dangerously dangling ('elf and safety clearly having the day off) and an underlying bustle which seemed to be enticing Christmas Day to come just a little bit quicker.

The foyer Christmas tree was huge, probably the biggest I'd ever seen. It made our moth-eaten charity shop offering, back at the three-storey town house, look a teeny bit insignificant. Actually, it was a great metaphor for just how I was feeling. Hospital huge and important. Red eyed mum tiny and insignificant.

Today was a day of huge significance. I took a deep breath and ushered my children in through the first set of sliding double doors.

I never got used to the feeling of entering the hospital. As the heat hit it was layered with an uncomfortable sensation, as if all the air was being sucked out of my lungs just as all the thoughts in my head dropped to the soles of my feet. Was it a combination of fear, hope and respect? Respect for the knowledge of all the people contained within, saving my son's life. It was also gratitude and humility. A powerful set of doors indeed.

The baubles on the tree were all blues and silvers and I used to joke with the children it was the grandest tree they would ever have in their entrance hall, for the hospital had become our home. Reluctantly I had begun to see those powerful doors as the entrance to our existence more than our Devon front door, its hideously peeling yellow paint was little more than a memory.

So much was hinging on today, Christmas Eve. We would find out if the treatment was working, if H had a chance at the rest of his life.

We walked the familiar route to the lifts, by-passing the wheelchairs. Today we were headed for the top floor, not Ward 34 on level five, to meet Dr John for an appointment on day beds, the outpatient ward for children with cancer and a ward which was always busy, even on Christmas Eve.

The lift stopped on level two and I cursed the opening of the doors. I just wanted to get it over with. In stepped one of the few doctors who actually wore a white coat, the Indian lady who was very direct. She was beaming. She must have great plans for Christmas. It took me a few moments to realise she was beaming at us.

Before my brain could engage with anything appropriate for the occasion – probably because I was so often in situations since arriving in Bristol when there was nothing appropriate for the occasion – she spoke.

'It's such good news. Don't tell Doctor John I told you,' she clearly couldn't contain herself. 'He'll tell you himself. But H is in remission!'

Two children looked up at me and saw my face break into a grin. Well, it made a change from tears. If grins were like Christmas trees mine was bigger than the one in the foyer.

Even though she should probably not have been having this conversation with me, in the lift, it didn't matter. H was in remission!

By the time we reached the seventh floor, it felt like Christmas. I'd been given the best Christmas present in the world. It was every Christmas present I'd ever had, wrapped up with every first kiss and every first step off a boat, a plane or a train to a new country.

'Christmas has arrived,' I said.

'We know that,' said H, 'we've been opening the advent calendars and Pops' been eating all the chocolate!'

Pops looked a bit guilty. 'But H didn't want it,' she said, looking at the floor.

Before I could say anything there was Dr John, beaming. We shuffled into the tiny office just round the corner from the reception desk and were ushered into regulation seats. Pops sat on my lap. I held her tightly.

I cannot remember what he said. When he uttered the words 'H', and 'in remission', in the same sentence, I couldn't stop grinning.

I knew we had a long way to go. I knew it was far from over. Remission did not mean all the leukaemia cells had been destroyed it just meant there weren't *too* many left. If subsequent rounds of chemo could kill off those remaining rogue cells – well, it was the big 'IF'.

As we left the tiny office, I knew H had had the best possible outcome to his first round of chemotherapy. One down, three to go. I knew it didn't mean we were a quarter of the way there, but it did mean we were headed in the right direction. It also meant there was every chance we could be home by Pops' birthday.

I think I hugged Dr John as we left. It was Merry Christmas all round.

We had to be back in hospital for December 28, to start the

second round of chemo. I was given strict instructions to stick to the rigid drug regime H was on – and to feed him up. I was even given an extra reel of feeding pipe fixing tape.

Every limb risking trip to the tiny Co-op round the back of the houses, every walk up the hill laden with bags stuffed full of M&S goodies, was going to be worth it. We had food, wine and presents galore even the fairy dust, thanks to Sandra, plus a knackered heating system which would (hopefully) ensure we would be toasty in the icy weather.

Back at the double doors by the enormous Christmas tree we were back in the real world. I could not risk walking up the hill back to the three-story town house because of all the ice. It was lethal. I just couldn't risk any of us falling over and breaking anything. I could also see H was very tired. I ordered yet another taxi to get us back to the house, he could never have walked up the hill.

I chivvied them along with the thought Hayley and her family were dropping in on their way up to Berkshire, if they could get through the weather, which was the worst Bristol had experienced since 1962.

As we waited for a taxi, I silently thanked everyone who had raised funds for CLIC Sargent, everyone who had ever walked a walk, danced a dance, sung, collected or organised an event for the charity. Knowing there were people out there who cared enough to give up their time to support complete strangers like us, meant so much.

I also thanked whoever had donated the Dr Who magazines to the waiting area in the foyer. It satisfied H and Pops for many hours over many months and was, in its own way, a little reminder of home.

As I walked over to the powerful doors yet again, to see if a taxi had pulled up, I looked over at both my children, dwarfed in such a huge space. H thin, pale and fragile. Pops looked tiny, dwarfed by everything around her. I already knew how difficult it would be for both of us to say goodbye on the evening of December 28. But the three of us would be together for the next four nights. And my son was in remission. Surely I could park the fear up somewhere else, just for a few days?

As a taxi pulled up, I resolved to do just that. It was Christmas Eve and it was time to celebrate with both my children and that was exactly what we were going to do. The three of us were going to have fun and eat ourselves silly. Worries about rocketing temperatures and having to call an ambulance, being iced in, the boiler failing, our own snow bound home back in Devon, the cats, money, work – worries about everything – had to be consigned to a bunker designed to hold worries and fears. They must be locked away in a place where even my frazzled brain could not access them. Surely we could be allowed to enjoy Christmas?

Seeing friends from Devon on Christmas Eve was special. We hadn't known the family for very long but they had braved the icy roads through Bristol to get to us and deliver all manner of gifts for the children, from so many people. Their boot seemed full of stuff just for us, including two huge boxes to add to the giant Christmas stocking made by H's school mates.

I made Hayley promise to text when they arrived at her mum's house. I had developed this odd foible of believing I, personally, was responsible for the safety of everyone who came to visit us. I felt if anyone had an accident on their way to, or from us, it would be my fault. I reasoned if they had not come to see us then they would not be on the roads and therefore not in any danger. I know it was odd but it was up there with the hospital room induced OCD, my obsession with an increasing collection of cloth bags (last count 27) and the belief one more special offer chocolate orange would ensure our food survival to the New Year.

In my defence extreme stress does strange things to the mind. It's never possible to have TOO many chocolate oranges – is it?

CHAPTER THIRTY-SIX

We were all set for Christmas Day. Just the three of us. My two children – hurrah, BOTH my children – and I. Cupboards full of food, fridge full of deliciousness, wine glasses to be filled and a truckload of presents to open. Thanks to the pound shops, markets and charity shops the house looked glorious. Even the front door looked festive, its red paint glowing with anticipation and a gaudy pound shop wreath enswathed with vintage baubles. Cards were hung, tinsel draped.

I'd even remembered a Christmas Radio Times. The telly was on and we watched, of course, 'The Snowman' and whatever other seasonal delights took our fancy. H was hooked up to his feeding machine, drugs administered.

The sheer pleasure of being in a living room with both my children, a sofa, glass in wine – I mean wine in glass – and a telly with a matching remote was a feeling I will never forget. My children, sofa, telly. Utter bliss.

At the appropriate hour we wrapped up well, crept into the front courtyard garden and scattered the fairy dust, not forgetting a very large carrot for Rudolf. It looked so wonderful on the white snow, by then very crisp and deep and even. In the centre of the courtyard was a Christmas tree their dad had delivered earlier in the day. A real tree. He'd driven through appalling weather just to get it to us. I'd hung big plastic glitter snowflakes on its bushy branches and it looked wonderful, particularly when it started snowing again.

We poured Sherry into a wine glass (Sherry glasses being in short supply in our current abode) and put an M&S mince pie on to a vintage plate (charity shop), placed them by the window in the first floor living room, which was, we agreed, the most sensible place in the absence of a chimney. We had magic on our side that night. Even now, when the three of us remember that Christmas Eve, it is remembered as 'a good 'un'.

I put the children to bed. They were so excited. We talked a bit.

'But will Father Christmas really know where we are this year,' Pops said. She was anxious he wouldn't be able to find us. I was anxious about her anxiety so everything was fine – no, really it was...

'It's OK Pops, I asked Becky to leave a note on our front door back home, just in case,' I said. How do we keep straight faces?

'But he'll know anyway,' said H, mustering an authority which surely came from his unswerving belief in the magic of Christmas. 'He'll know where we are Pops, he will. He always does.'

Did I feel guilty about the lie? Of course I didn't.

For those few hours that Christmas Eve we were the 21st century Dickensian family – divorced single mum of two sat round an artificial Christmas Tree, Tiny Tim's crutch evident in H's feeding tube and wiggly, the last of the bank account cleared out by M&S goose fat roast potatoes, the snow-covered Bristol skyline an evocative urban landmark as striking as any London view or *Christmas Carol* film set.

I went back to the living room, safe in the knowledge the house was toasty warm, locked up and the curtains were drawn.

Had I drawn around me the very curtains Dickens hung about Scrooge's four poster on that fictional Victorian Christmas Eve, my mood could not have plummeted faster.

As I sat on the expensive Next sofa, I began to feel edgy, uncomfortable. I had barely managed a single glass of red and I couldn't concentrate on the TV screen.

My head hurt, so I took some Paracetamol. I felt a vague sense of tightness under my left boob. I tried to ignore it. But the more I tried to ignore it, the more it hurt. I began to feel sick. It wasn't that 'sick-with-fear' kind of feeling. I really wanted to throw up, but then I realised I couldn't even get to the bathroom and it was only a few steps away. What on earth was going on?

I thought if I could get off the sofa and lie on the floor, I'd feel better.

I got off the sofa and lay on the floor. I didn't feel any better.

I lay there, looking up at the ceiling and the pain took hold. I felt as if my insides were being dragged out through a small hole on the left of my chest.

I thought I'd go and get some water from the kitchen, but I could barely move.

I lay there, trying to keep my breathing calm and frantically trying to work out what on earth was happening.

Finally, I figured, the stress was catching up with me. That was it. Stress. And it wasn't really surprising, was it?

My mothering mind was racing. The stockings were filled and I'd stashed them in the secret under stair cupboard on the floor below. Check. Oh this pain – go away! It wouldn't. I may as well have been visited by ghosts – in fact, bring on those ghosts they'd be less scary than the pain.

Bed, get to bed, said brain – Inner Goddess had clearly buggered off for Christmas. Thanks for that love!

I shelved the water idea and crawled up the stairs, dragged myself across the top bedroom carpet and rolled onto the mattress on the floor we had made up earlier for me. Both my children were fast asleep in the two beds, the gentle click click click of H's food pump a strangely soothing sound.

My head was pounding, the pain seemed worse. Bring me ghosts – please.

I felt exhausted, my body heavy.

'OHMYGOD I'm having a heart attack.'

Had-to-think-clearly. Must get help. Can't wake children they will be frightened.

OHMYGOD the children. I can't have a heart attack – who will look after my children? It's Christmas FORGODSAKE. What if I die and they find my body in the morning? I felt the tears forcing their way out of my closed eyelids.

'Please don't let me die just yet. If I die and ... and... and then what happens to Pops?'

I was being visited by ghosts and they were bastards.

Breathe and think.

Be calm.

Think.

OK. No pain in my left arm, definitely no pain in my left arm. That's good. That's very good. Phone; call for an ambulance. Can't. Phone downstairs. Down downstairs in kitchen. I can't do two flights of stairs. Have to, don't want to die. Have to look after my children.

In the end, the pain and exhaustion must have knocked me out.

I slept for several hours because when I woke up – yes, I woke up! - there was light coming in through the bedroom curtains. I heard the click click click of H's feeding pump. They were both fast asleep.

Merry Christmas world! I'm alive. I wanted to throw the

windows open just like Scrooge had. I wanted to dance with the world and cook the biggest goose I'd never seen.

Then I remembered my son had cancer

I crawled out of bed, crept down two flights of stairs retrieved the stockings and laid them out in the living room. I even remembered to sprinkle the secret glitter stash all over the window sill.

I have no idea what happened that night but suspect it was a combination of indigestion (from which I'd never suffered), stress and the fear of daring to relax.

I have told the story to friends several times since and we all laugh – it's the way I tell 'em...

I knew, if I carried on living with this level of fear and stress, there was nothing to say I wouldn't have a heart attack.

But for now, I was alive and so were both my children.

And it was Christmas Day.

CHAPTER THIRTY-SEVEN

It was probably the absence of the timed click click click of H's feeding machine which woke me up for a second time.

I lay there, grateful to be alive, my mind numb with exhaustion. My Christmas Wish - five minutes of silence - was magically granted.

After a while I heard both H and Pops stirring.

'H, are you awake?' said Pops.

Followed by H's. 'Do you think he's been?'

'Shall we go and have a look?' said Pops.

'Shhh, don't wake mummy' said H.

It had become second nature for H to be aware of his feeding tube. If he wasn't, he was in danger of dislodging it out of his stomach and watching it snake out of his nose, all the while knowing just how hideous it would be to feed it back in. I think it was the fear of it all which made him so aware.

Watching them through half closed eyes I saw H gingerly pick up the stand which held all the paraphernalia as the pair made their way down to the first floor living room.

As I rolled out of bed to follow them, I realised I was fully dressed. Thank goodness neither of them had seen. They would immediately have known something was wrong. I changed into pyjamas. What a topsy-turvy life this was!

By the doorway of the living room, I watched as they poked and prodded, marvelled at the glitter and made comments like 'Ooooh you've got a...'

'No, don't say it, I want to find it myself...'

'What's that then?'

'I don't know yet; I haven't opened it'.

'Shall we eat some chocolate?'

It was such fun to watch and listen. I even forgot for a bit where we were.

'How about I make a coffee, you two have some juice and then we can open your stockings,' I said to two very excited little beings.

It was the start of a wonderful, wonderful day.

One of the best I have ever had with my children.

It was everything every child should have at Christmas – ripping wrapping paper off presents, playing with new stuff, tearing open packets, laughing, giggling, bickering and eating and drinking whatever they wanted. Although H was far choosier than normal, he did brilliantly and I was confident enough to knock out his lunchtime feed, which gave him so much more freedom.

People rang to wish us Happy Christmas. I cooked a full Christmas dinner (why had I never used these pre done goose wotsit potatoes in disposable foil trays before?), drank decent wine, ate far too much chocolate and we all hunkered down to watch seasonal offerings on telly, all punctuated with plenty of naps.

The day had been created out of nothing. I was so, so grateful to everyone who had made it possible, particularly to H's and Pops' primary school.

H's giant stocking was like the stuff of dreams, and I was

thrilled he had the energy to rip the paper off so many presents. Pops kept pace with her brother and thanks to the kindness of the teachers, I had all sorts to open as well.

Of course I cried. I was so touched.

'We know that,' sniggered Inner Goddess, who seemed to have woken up.

The two huge boxes contained two giant fluffy Dulux dogs. We three laughed our socks off.

We had a call from our friends in Reading, who had been due to spend Boxing Day with us. The roads were impassable in places, so we agreed it was not safe enough for them to even think of attempting such a trip.

It meant we had 48 hours in pyjamas. The snow had done its bit to wrap us up in a bubble all of our own. Turkey sandwich anyone?

CHAPTER THIRTY-EIGHT

THE ANALOGY WASN'T LOST ON ME: ROUND TWO. WE WERE IN A BOXING ring except today the boxing promoter hadn't showed up to sort out the fight.

Should one talk about cancer in terms of a fight, good versus evil? I did not for a moment feel I was fighting an enemy; I don't like war even when it is spoken of in a different context. What we were fighting for – what I was fighting for - was survival, physical and emotional.

There is no win or lose with cancer. Diagnosis means treatment and treatment leads to respite. Respite – remission – means you carry on living in a way that is treatment and cancer free; hopefully. But remission doesn't mean you are cured. Cancer is complicated and so is the language around it. This I was learning. Nothing to do with cancer is straightforward. This I was also learning.

I rang the evening of the day before we were due back to be told yes, there should be a bed available, but if there wasn't, they would put us in Ward 35.

No thanks, I said, we don't want to go into Ward 35, the ward with a gruesome kitchen, sofas even dirtier than the small secret 'family room' tucked away on the Ward 34 entrance corridor. A ward we didn't know and a ward, rumour had it, full of teenagers not all of whom were fighting cancer. Ward 35 had become, in my head, a place to be avoided. I had often seen two young women outside the front entrance, dressed in *'Primani'* pyjamas (of course by then I knew all about every garment *'Primani'* was shipping in from sweat shops, to make a few people at the top of the feeding chain richer; I was guilty of supporting the cheap clothing bonanza).

'Primani' pyjamas, grubby furry slippers, dyed hair, chain smoking and a wild look in the eye; *'I'm different to you but I can handle it'* syndrome. I'd seen that look before, in another hospital where I was a hospital radio DJ. We only got requests from the patients on ward 12, who were let out during 'windows in their medication'. I'd also seen 'the look' in the eyes of men and women living in the elderly hospital wards where I volunteered as a teenager. Men and women staring, the usual filters on life absent because the balance of the mind had slipped; dementia, fear, mental illness, a stroke, every stare silently said, 'get me out of here'.

There was nothing to say I wasn't developing 'the look'. I even had the *'Primani'* pyjamas to go with it, though I had chosen pyjama bottoms with blue and white stripes which made me look more like a convict.

I did not want to enter Ward 35. I knew some of those filter-less youngsters were being treated on Ward 35 and I did not want to be there with my children. We wouldn't know anybody there. Would the people there understand about keeping things clean? Would the paperwork follow us or would vital drugs information be lost by different staff who had no idea what H had already endured? Would their regimes be different from Ward 34?

Ward 34 had become our home, despite the torture inflicted. Ironically Ward 34 had become a place of safety for us. How had the fear turned so quickly into familiarity? How was it possible that in this half-life of an existence, we had been able to form such an attachment to this hospital ward?

No doubt a psychologist would find it easy to explain. We had been plucked from our Devon home, lost almost everything we had known and the closest we had to a 'home' was a space which had two beds and two sinks in it. On Ward 34 we knew the people, the routines, where the corridors went, which toilet had a dodgy lock, where the sluice room was, how to procure non latex purple gloves, where cardboard pooh, wee and sick receptacles were stacked. I wasn't giving up on Ward 34 without a fight. Oh Lordy – fighting again...

I packed for me and H to return to hospital the following day. Mum and dad were staying for two more nights, when Cousin Debbie and her sister Terry were due, until Magda was able to get from Jersey to Bristol.

That evening, sitting quietly in the living room with my mum, I tried to calm her down.

'I put it down, over there on that table and he moved it. And now he doesn't know where it is and I can't find it either,' said mum, getting more and more wound up about losing her book.

'Let me get you a glass of wine,' I said, 'and I'll see if I can find it.'

'But I've looked in the kitchen and it's not there,' she retorted. 'And I don't want a glass of wine. I just want to read my book. Is that too much to ask? He's getting worse. You don't know how hard this is for me.'

'Look mum,' I said, 'dad is not in a very good place. But what do you want me to do about it? You say he doesn't need any more tests. I think he does. You refuse to make another appointment with the GP and I can't do that for you because you won't let me. I'm stuck in Bristol Mum. This is hard for both of us. You know I think it's Alzheimer's or early onset dementia or something...'

'Well he's already had tests and the doctor says it isn't. He passed all the tests,' said mum, becoming even more defensive.

'But mum, things have got worse. Even I can see that in the time since you were here last month. Dad's not well.'

'I can't deal with that now,' said mum, in a way which clearly said the conversation was over.

Life is full of pecking orders. Seen and unseen, heeded and unheeded.

Whether I liked it or not mum had to look out for my dad while I was in Bristol, and I had to look out for H and Pops.

Neither mum nor my brother wanted to accept how ill dad was. All the while they remained in denial there was little anyone else could do. I had one battle on my hands (that bloody word again). I knew I could not fight (fight!) dad's corner as well. It made me so incredibly sad.

I found mum's book downstairs. I carried it up to the living room, dad came out of the shower, dressed in his customary cloud of aftershave – yes, and trousers.

I saw his eyes light up at the glass of red in my hand.

'Fancy a glass dad?' I said.

He grinned at me and nodded but said nothing. I think he really couldn't find the words he wanted so he stood, a puzzled look on his face.

Then he saw mum's book.

'I was looking for that,' he said, and grinned at me before shuffling into the living room to join her.

I slept fitfully, trying not to worry about H. I was concerned about my parents. And I was dreading leaving Pops tomorrow.

As it happened, we had a 24-hour reprieve, which at the time really pissed me off. One more day in limbo meant a day further away from home.

Looking back, it was the last day I ever really spent with my dad. Dad as I actually remembered him. And for that I remain incredibly grateful.

H and I could not return to Ward 34 because there had been an outbreak of sickness and diarrhoea, so the ward was being deep cleaned.

The nurse I spoke to assured me all would be well. She was fairly sure there would be a bed for us, on Ward 34, the following day.

You learn with hospitals nothing is certain, nothing is set in stone. What you are told one day, can be completely different the next and it's not anybody's fault. Illness and disease are as unpredictable as the weather and there's no such thing as an NHS clairvoyant.

Mum came for a walk with the three of us. Dad stayed at home for a nap after lunch. Enough of the icy slush had melted so we could walk on solid pavement.

The air was cold and very crisp. We wrapped up with bright new hats, scarves and gloves. The road we found ourselves living in harked back to grander days with large three storey town houses, extravagant front doorways, huge Georgian windows and plenty of original features gracing entrances, ornate railings enclosing charming front gardens. Everywhere was festooned with Christmas wreaths, twinkling fairy lights and festive creativity proclaiming a winter holiday in full swing.

The sun was low, the pavements crisp and many of the facades were bathed in a golden glow more befitting a woodland clearing than an urban forest of hard brick lines, chiselled stone pillars and fancy chimneys reaching for the sky. As the light faded further, I could see moving tableaux playing out in front rooms, Christmas tree lights of every shape and hue framing family gatherings, contentment descending.

As we got to the end of the very long road it became a square surrounded by even bigger, grander houses in varying states of repair, most with an overall feel of faded elegance.

It was getting cold. I realised we were almost outside CLIC House, the home-from-home refuge funded by CLIC Sargent. The place Pops and I were supposed to have stayed in those first few nights. It was the house Pops and Magda would be moving to in the New Year.

I couldn't resist looking in through some of the windows so we wandered up one of the driveways. The house had been two, now knocked into one. We found ourselves looking in to a very large, high-ceilinged living room graced with mismatching furniture and a huge Christmas tree, decorated with an eclectic mix never destined to appear in a glossy magazine. And a family to go with it. I vaguely recognised them from the ward and, not wanting to intrude, knowing how precious those snatched moments of family togetherness were, we withdrew. We were on the outside, looking in.

It was time to go home. 'Home'; a strange notion. We had a cosy place to return to, dripping with Christmas fripperies. And plenty of *Branston* to go with cold turkey, ham and, if I was lucky, a bit of smoked salmon.

We all watched telly that evening. It was as normal as normal gets. Even an argument with mum, telling her to lay off dad, who insisted on following her around from room to room. I could appreciate why it was so annoying but he was confused, he didn't know the house and he must have wondered why we were there. He couldn't even read H and Pops a bedtime story. I was happy to have spent a bit of time with dad, and we'd had a few laughs.

'Another Sherry Dad?' I said. He grinned at me, the ends of his overgrown eyebrows wiggling in agreement.

'Don't you think you two have had enough already?' said mum, disapproval seeping out of her pores.

Me and my dad giggled like naughty school kids who had raided the grown-up's drinks cabinet.

I rang Ward 34 to find out if they could tell me if we had a bed tomorrow or not. It was another 'call us back in the morning when we should know for sure'.

Bags packed, drugs administered, last feed given; I read to H and Pops.

I was dreading the next few weeks, but it would bring us closer to home. It was the only way I could look at the impending separation from Pops. We were in the loop and there was no escape.

Bloody cancer.

CHAPTER THIRTY-NINE

We had a bed on Ward 34, said the nurse down the phone the following morning. 'On the ward', she added, *'on the bay'*.

Dismiss all thoughts of Miami beach-front houses where an early morning stroll entails white silky sand bathing your toes in a luxuriously invigorating spa like treatment, before a dip in the sparkling blue. Followed by a peachy iced tea. Oh no!

'On the bay' meant one of the five beds in a large room round the back of the wall where the nurses' station was. *'On the bay'* meant you were sharing your air and sinks and toilets and flooring and taps and everything with everybody else on the ward. You were sharing with anybody and everybody who traipsed through the airless space.

From cleaners and auxiliary staff to the wheels of the trolleys which had rolled goodness knows where. All the bottoms of the shoes of each doctor, nurse, porter, kitchen assistant, teacher, play therapist, story teller, student, volunteer, consultant and every single visitor to all the other patients who had the misfortune to also be *'on the bay'*.

We were now in hazardous territory. The toilets were communal. Every small child or sibling who came to visit and wiped their poo or splashed their wee somewhere it shouldn't, was a risk for H. It soon became clear some adults had yet to learn how to use a toilet; yes, I do mean flushing after a number two. In a high dependency children's oncology ward, cleanliness could mean the difference between contracting a life-threatening infection and dying or living. Well, you can see where I'm coming from. For those of you who may feel I had become a drama queen since arriving in Bristol, reading on may give a different perspective.

It also meant we had gone from a prison cell existence to the big, wide open prairie-like space of a very busy hospital ward: with people.

Cancer is a contrary beast. It is complex and therefore the way it is treated has to be multi-layered. The way you treat one cancer is different from the way you treat another. Ward 34 patients were at different stages of their treatments. Some had immune systems working, others didn't.

It would have been impossible to 'police' all visitors arriving on the ward. If someone had a cold it didn't matter, they were visiting a patient in for a blood transfusion or a morning's chemo. How would they know the patient on the next bed was vulnerable to the sneezed-out snot showering a bedside table on wheels? Did it matter someone used a tap on the sink by the far wall and left vomit residues on the tap? Not to a patient in for a night observation. But those lurking bugs could be fatal to Tiny Chap over by the window in the far corner.

I knew how two of the consultants felt about five beds in one space because I asked them. They believed the oncology patients should be nursed in isolation, for each patient's safety. But you cannot design an entire hospital around one select group of patients when space and money are limited.

It was a bug lottery *'on the bay'*. I hated it on sight.

I made myself think of the advantages. Now we had access to 'other people'. H might make a friend. I would get the chance to compare notes with other parents, share the experience. By that I mean share the fear. I knew no one else could share our experience, even by child cancer wards standards it was shaping up to be unique. It didn't take long to discover how terrified other parents had been when they found out there was a swine flu family being treated on the ward. Our flu could have killed their child.

It was almost a New Year. The residues of a hospital Christmas were lingering on two tables pushed together in front of the glass double doors, facing a walk through from one side of the hospital to another. Doors we were never supposed to open.

On the tables were opened boxes of chocolates, only the blue wrappered toffees left. Half-eaten packets of biscuits, all the chocolate ones gone. A token fruit bowl. A few Twiglets in the bottom of a cardboard 'party' drum. Crumbs, flat packets and brown plastic cake trays – minus the cakes – mocked the near empty tin of 'luxury shortbread' vying for space with a pile of broken cheese straws and a squashed vanilla fondant fancy.

As the nurse walked us past the carnage of boredom, I wanted to run and when I saw H's disappointment at the promised feast of naughtiness, I felt too weary to run. Running not allowed.

'Hey, we've got a bed in the corner' I said to H, trying to chivvy him along. 'And we've got a window! I reckon Bed 9 is the best bed of the lot,' I whispered.

He smiled; his pale head framed by the weird line of stubby dark hairs clinging on for dear life.

It was not lost on either of us that there was no telly by the bed, not even a bedside table.

We plonked our bags down and sat on his new bed, legs dangling over the sides, the hospital corners standing to attention.

'Well, we made it back to Ward 34,' I said, H's look telling me that was not a positive.

'When this one is over, we're even closer to getting back home.' I was trying to find reasons to be cheerful (part two!) I was failing. Why don't you get back into bed... (oops, showing my age. Wonder how Ian Dury had coped with all his time in hospital?).

'Come on love, let's get your quilt on the bed. Do you want to put your pyjamas on?'

The scowl, which would have made a teenager proud, said he didn't.

Then it was all bustle and false bonhomie.

'You've missed the party,' said the nurse, 'but there's New Year to come yet. That's always fun here.'

I didn't believe her. Fun? Yes of course I felt patronised. If it was so much 'fun' how come so many of the regular nurses weren't around and it was staff from other wards? How is being trapped in hospital, with a nine-year old who has cancer 'fun', at any time of the year?

It was back to temperature, blood pressure and finding a drip stand. It was back to hideous drugs and sick and pooh and card-board pee bottles and the shitty sluice room and getting on with making out to the outside world that yes, everything's fine. When it wasn't. It was back to being scared. Except now I felt fear every time someone sneezed, every time a stranger walked in to the ward – and there were a lot. Where had they been? What was on the bottom of their shoes? Had they washed their hands?

It was also back to a pull-down bed. And I had yet to experience the braless morning shuffle in pyjamas to the communal shower round the corner, dodging cliques of docs and walking back head in towel clutching toilet bag hoping I hadn't left anything behind, hoping nothing was on show that shouldn't be.

Get a grip said Inner Goddess. Stop mind whinging and get on with it!

'Come on H, let's see if we can find a telly that works. And let's choose some DVDs!'

It emerged just how bad the state of TVs was on the ward. No one seemed interested in sorting them out, because of the impending digital switch over. The hospital management was looking at different ways of providing screens for patients. We had hit the facility desert, the gap in provision. If finding gaps in provision – holes in nets – was an art form, we always hit the jackpot. I'd been darn good at it for a number of years. Outside in.

In the meantime, it was every family for themselves. I was told by the ward's housekeeper even when new TVs were provided, they often went missing.

'What, people steal them?' I said, unable to get my head round the idea people would steal from a children's cancer ward.

'Actually, you need to watch all your stuff in here,' a nurse told me, 'things go missing and we can't be responsible. Don't leave anything valuable *on the bay*.'

Great, couldn't even leave my handbag by the bed. Oh for the sanctuary of a room all to ourselves. The irony of not realising just how lucky we had been to be nursed in isolation, getting a room to ourselves, was suddenly quite hilarious. There had been me, wanting contact with other people. Now we had it and, well, be careful what you wish for!

Thefts, on a children's cancer ward? Now that really is sick.

'Get a grip', said Inner Goddess. *'Just get on with it!'*.

The bay had five beds. Two on the long left wall as you walked in, two at the short end, closely packed, the one by the window being ours. The last one was in the opposite corner to us, sandwiched between the outside wall and the communal toilet/bathroom, conveniently located by the corridor to freedom, leading out of the ward, past the tiny and imperfectly formed parents' kitchen.

I noted, with huge relief, the spot so close to ours was occupied by a boy called Sam, who also had AML. I'd spoken to his parents in the parents' kitchen, post swine flu. I recognised the handmade sea themed patchwork quilt adorning the bed - another patchwork quilt! I'd seen it and commented on it, after spotting it through the small oblong (from the outside) of reinforced glass on the door of Room 3, where doctors had saved Sam's life. He had been close to death when he was admitted. The leukaemia stole the sight of an eye. No one knew if the loss would be permanent.

It was his mum, Tam, who had been the first person to give me a hug since the nightmare began. She had proved to be the most beautiful and kind woman anyone could ever meet. She cooked proper food which smelt great, had very long hair in a plait, came from Cornwall, wore funky handmade boots and made stuff.

I knew she had two sons – three-year old Sam and his younger brother, fourteen-month Ollie. She had a partner who was their dad. Her mum was also with them in Bristol. A close-knit family, I thought.

Tam's family arrived almost a month after us and were living in the CLIC House annexe with another family, who were also on the ward. I couldn't remember their names. Their son was also being treated for AML. Staff said how unusual it was to have three at once. Don't mention buses, it's not funny. He was in the bed out on a limb, in the opposite corner beside the communal bathroom. I'd talked to his mum and dad a few times as they took solace by the front entrance, puffing harder than the wide-eyed teenagers.

Sam and his family were out. He was coming to the end of his first round of chemo. Hope Tam didn't mind my snoring.

I loved the funky fairy lights she'd draped on the curtain rail, the little bedside lamp on the cabinet on wheels. Tam would be clean. Tam would be responsible. It would be OK.

'*Yes*', said Inner Goddess, *'all will be well'*.

We explored our new 'home'. I realised when the pull-down bed was down there was no space between it, and H's bed. Funny that. I had been told when we arrived the reason Pops couldn't stay with us was because there was no room. Doctors and nurses had to have access to both sides of the bed, in case there was an emergency. So, what happens *'on the bay'* if there was a problem? '*Oh, just don't go there*', said Irritated Inner One. *'Just bloody well get on with it – and with good grace please. Thank you very much'*.

H and I found a telly. But we couldn't make it work.

Dad of patient in bed by long wall wandered over.

'They're all pretty knackered in here,' he said, helpfully. 'Has it got an adapter, that little silver thing?' he said.

'Erm,' came my blank reply.

'Don't worry, I'll find you one. The housekeeper's got a box of stuff and there's usually some in there.' Techy Husbands are everywhere!

I mumbled about him being very kind. He got the telly working.

We got chatting. They were a young couple, mid-twenties, from Bristol. Their son had developed difficulty walking, several months before. Repeated visits to their GP had been unhelpful.

He was six or seven and when he was unable to walk – yes, unable to walk at all, he'd been sent for X-rays. How crap is that! Mind you, we'd gone from swine flu to leukaemia in one painful leap.

It reinforced my view even doctors do not embrace childhood cancer. It is so unusual, why would they? What GP is on the lookout for it, how much does it feature on a medical syllabus? I'd seen the fear in the eyes of the young doctor in Torbay Hospital. Childhood cancer is not 'out there'.

The hospital had discovered a lump on his spine. Surgery gave him back some mobility but opened the door to months and months of uncertainty and chemotherapy. It was not a straight forward cancer. There seemed to be no clear treatment path. Doctors hadn't seen it that way before. I realised I was asking far too many questions and tried to pull back, but they clearly wanted – needed? – to talk.

They would have to go through several more rounds of chemo before the doctors could test for the state of the cancer, before anyone would know what the future might hold. He was their only son, the only grandchild in a large extended Bristol family.

His mother stayed with him at night. She would curl round him on his bed as he slept, as if trying to protect him any way she could. How they both slept on the raised hospital bed I have no idea. It was heart breaking at night, to see Dad, who stayed as late as he could, leaving them both behind. He wasn't allowed to stay and he had to work, full-time. The separation must have been so very hard for them.

She wore tight pink tee shirts with mindless statements like 'cats heart pink' and 'shoes are for life'. She clearly loved sequins and fake nails, which matched the blonde streaked hair. Apart from our sons having cancer we had virtually nothing in common. Well, apart from the sequins.

I was so glad we had arrived on the ward in plenty of time to hang around doing absolutely nothing for several hours, until the chemo drugs eventually arrived in their blue plastic tray.

'Be nice,' said Inner Irritating One. If I'd known how often she'd have to give me a talking to during round two, I'd probably have throttled her.

Again, I had those helpless feelings. '*Oh go on then. Fill my son with poison, make him as sick as you possibly can. Then, when he gets better, let's start all over'.*

Some mum I am. I'm the one supposed to be keeping my child safe and healthy. I didn't wish I had cancer, but if it had been me, I could have taken the hit. I felt adrift in the sea of motherhood, the world of upside down. A place that simply shouldn't be.

I just wanted to cry. Then cry some more. Instead, I got out the sewing bag and for a while H and I sewed as the drugs ticked away, filling his veins and tubes with stuff so toxic it could probably destroy an Indian hotel's worth of cockroaches.

'Do you want to watch a film mum?' said H.

'Go on then, what do you fancy?'

Our foray to the DVD 'library', H pushing his drip stand, was a waste of time. The DVD player on the telly didn't work.

H dozed, I started cleaning the over-the-bed table with antibacterial wipes and cleaned out his bedside trolley on wheels, the one I'd had to hunt down from somewhere else.

Every passing member of staff we asked about a new telly couldn't help. I did get the look from a couple of them 'we're trying to save lives here you know...'

My silent reproach *'and yeah, cancer's even shittier without a telly'* fell on deaf minds.

'Pops will be here soon,' I said.

She duly arrived, accompanied by mum and dad. My daughter was clingy and wouldn't leave my lap. Mum was clearly not enjoying the lovely ward experience and dad sat in a chair, dozing, not really part of anything.

'It's fine mum. Why don't you all go and you can get your tea started.'

She didn't need asking twice. I walked them all to the front entrance of the hospital, the enormous Christmas tree still sparkling away.

I watched my daughter as she walked up the road. If it was physically possible to feel your heart break in two, then that's what I felt by the outside automatic double doors of Bristol Children's Hospital. Again.

I kept telling myself this was temporary, we had to go through this to get H well, that it was a small price to pay so H could live.

By the time Inner Irritator had started and I'd told her to 'PISS OFF', tears were streaming down my face and I had to go to the second-floor loos for toilet paper and a face wash with cold water.

If schizophrenia was an art form, I was getting pretty good at it. Back on the ward I had to smile. My face was so taught you'd think I'd had Botox.

CHAPTER FORTY

We three had obviously relaxed over Christmas, despite the rather large family gathering of thirteen I ended up hosting at Charly's House the day before we came back into hospital. My brother and his girlfriend had a row, because he refused to be in a family photograph. But apart from that it was fine.

The blog summed up the contrast in our change of circumstances; cosy family Christmas to paediatric oncology in one short taxi ride. It's not that I'd forgotten the intensity of it all, of course I hadn't. But the contrast between having our own room and an open ward was quite stark.

I blogged the day after we arrived back:

'Living on a hospital ward, surrounded by other very sick children and their families, is akin to the old-fashioned images and sounds of Bedlam...it is distressing...

'Earlier this evening I walked Pops back to our accommodation (which at one point today we were told we had to be out of by 8am tomorrow!!! I don't think so....) settled her in with mum and dad and then walked back to the hospital where H was waiting for me. I couldn't actually get in the ward because a five-year old was throwing an almighty eppy, repeatedly crashing his drip stand into the door

screaming out all sorts ... Managed to get in, but the little chap had clearly sent disturbed vibes out amongst the troops generally... I burst into tears because I'd just had to say goodbye to a crying Pops. Yet again. This separation thing is so tough. Am learning more about other family stories ...

'Anyways, couple of hours later and all quiet on the Western front. Eppy child removed to a side room where he eventually stopped because he had exhausted himself. Small baby crying had obviously fallen asleep. Terminally ill toddler in pain finally sedated and teeny tumour chap settled after the trauma of eppy child had clearly left him upset. H being amazing, his gifted MP3 player, full of witch stories, helped dull out the wails, screams and shouts of the other patients.

'Lights off, lovely and peaceful, chemo drugs pumping away silently when bone cancer kiddie returns to ward at 9.15pm and mum promptly puts all the lights on. Terminal toddler woken up, teeny tumour chap disturbed and H, who was drifting off, comes to and is forced to listen to inane 'Mr Bean' DVD piped out of bone cancer patient's telly because Mum seems to think as long as she gets her own child off to sleep, it really doesn't matter about anyone else's child... When lovely nurse asked her to turn it down, she gets a load of cheek from bone cancer child who thinks it's 'mean' to be told to turn it down. He's five years old. Mum carries on flicking through, very loudly, crap mag and I can still hear 'Mr Bean' through the curtain.

'Can I make judgements about other people's parenting in such extreme situations? Just want to get out of here... But have to put up and shut up...I guess that's all the other parents are trying to do, any way they can...'

One of the nurses told me eppy child's behaviour was not unusual. They let them tantrum, to get it out of their system, she said. In many ways it is the only way a small child can relieve their frustration, find an antidote to the pain and discomfort of hideous processes.

Met a mum in the parents' kitchen earlier today. Her daughter was about fifteen months and had been in Ward 34 most of her life, having been diagnosed with a brain tumour at six weeks old. If her parents had refused the treatment, they could have been taken to court by the hospital authorities, the treatment forcibly given. I got the feeling, from the conversation, all treatments would do little to prolong such a young life for much longer. It was heart breaking and cruel.

I was wandering around a minefield of moral issues. My new favourite mug was emblazoned with 'Keep Calm and Carry On'. Sandra found one which said, 'Now Panic and Freak Out'. Maybe I had the wrong mug?

CHAPTER
FORTY-ONE

THERE WAS A BUZZ OF EXCITEMENT OUT THERE, OUT THERE IN THE REAL world. I must have picked it up from the BBC News page, my 'home page' on laptop. Not only was it working but the bed head, the space-age control panel with all its' switches and outlets and plug-in bits, had an internet lead socket.

If you indulged in a bit of acrobatics, using the bright red cable acquired from the education department, I could plug the laptop in to a socket on the wall by the window. The red lead reached its own socket – if it was strung across the top of H's bed - thus allowing me to use said shiny black laptop. I strongly suspect the 'health and safety' department would have had something to say about the intricate wiring set up, which looked like the early stages of a giant spider's lair. A poisonous lair! By the time I was plugging in, it was lights out on the ward (around 10pm), evening vitals had been checked and H was just about beginning to bed down for the night.

One hoped all the others were too. It's hard to go from your own bedroom where you are alone, to a small clinical room where people are free to come and go as they please. It was even worse on the ward, where you didn't even have enough privacy to fart. At least by then I knew I wasn't the only snorer.

Once H was asleep, I was free to surf away. It helped to shut everything else out. I had managed to cannibalise some earphones from a bag of mobile phone stuff Kate had lent me. BBC iPlayer et al were invaluable. It also felt a bit like being eight again, when I was secretly reading Enid Blyton under the bed covers, using a torch.

'Is your light out yet?' mum would holler up the stairs.

'Yes mum,' I could answer in all honesty. I only got rumbled when dad noticed the household battery supply was diminishing, with no logical explanation...

It's not that 'calm' would descend on the ward when the lights went out. Even at night it wasn't 'calm'. As parents or carers, we were all on high alert. You knew even when you did fall asleep, invariably you'd get woken up by the noises of illness. Especially such intense illness, such 24-hour, full on illness, with so much ministering by so many.

Funny how illness lived out in hospital is such a noisy beast. From nurses doing their checks, the clicking of the medicine pumps, feeding pumps, oxygen machines, nocturnal doctors' rounds, other laptops and TVs humming away, the coughing, vague voices floating around from the nurses' station, someone's squeaky shoes as they carried a poo filled cardboard bed pan to the sluice room, a flushing toilet, muffled mobile phone conversations, a shattered parent risking a 2am shower. The rustle of crisp packets, the crunching of Crunchies. One night it was two staff flirting round the corner.

I could have got used to the firemen though. Well, it's not often you get a bunch of firemen (collective noun 'a flare of firemen'?) strolling into your 'bedroom', in full uniform and there's you in your flimsy nightie, hanging around wondering why the alarm is going this time, not quite needing to be rescued... I categorically deny I kept burning toast in the kitchen. No, I absolutely did not, Your Honour. Tempting though it might have been. I'd clearly been on my own for far too long. I knew I had. I knew that before Bristol.

But no, it wasn't the firemen who created the buzz of excitement, (Well, they did, but that's another book, surely...). It was the impending 'Blue Moon'. And it was due to make an appearance on New Year's Eve.

Now, if you have to spend New Year's Eve in hospital with a sick boy and a distraught daughter up the road, then you may as well have the pleasure of something special. A 'Blue Moon' is a moon so called because it will be the second lunar scenario in one calendar month. It is said you may make a wish on one and its special powers will bathe you in good luck for, well, many moons to come. Elvis, Ella Fitzgerald, and Sinatra – they all thought 'Blue Moons' were pretty special too!

It's a no-brainer what I wished for.

I even got special permission to bring a bottle of Cava in to the ward that night. Lovely Zoe and Chemical Ken were doing their best to imbue the ward with a bit of party spirit and a few nice nibbles, which I added to, in the hope people would join in.

I had a real bee in my bonnet about having Pops with us that night. It was agreed she was allowed to stay until midnight, and then I would have to take her back to Charly's House, where mum and dad were staying until my cousins could get to Bristol. It was not ideal, and certainly not great for a seven-year-old to be up so late, but it was a small victory. Why she could not have been allowed to stay the night on the ward, which was almost empty as most patients had been sprung for the occasion, I do not know. I booked a taxi for half past midnight, so I could get her back to Charly's House safely.

The three of us watched a film and indulged in yet another M&S ready meal (beef casserole and buttery mash was on special). H ate most of the green vegetables but no beef or mash, Pops just wanted the mash (she's 'allergic' to casseroles because they have 'bits' in them and she is deeply suspicious of onions) so I ended up with most of the beef which, in all honesty, needed a robust red to help wash it down...

There was a funny vibe on the ward. Of course I don't mean funny hilarious. There is always something a bit uncomfortable about institutional places where faceless people are trying so hard to inject a bit of 'bonhomie', when there really is none to be found. An invite had gone out to Ward 35 in case anyone wanted to join 'the party'.

The large white 'ward board' listing who was in, who their consultant was, when they were due to be sprung was not very helpful. I didn't really know anyone and the other 'regular' bed just wanted to hunker down, forget where they were. I so should have done the same.

Yet driven by some inane 'it's the New Year therefore you have to celebrate' ethos – something I had suffered from for years – I had to mark the occasion. It felt like I had to 'celebrate' the impending year, look towards a good future by shutting out the crap of the last one, of which there was, undeniably, quite a bit.

Celebrating the New Year was something I didn't actually want to be doing. A 'party' was the last thing I felt like. What was I actually celebrating? In reality there was no actual party because everyone else was so much more sensible than me.

I was looking towards a future which may or may not have H in it, several more months of hideous treatment and uncertainty, no one to share it with (as in 'significant other') and I certainly wasn't going to get glammed up in the hope I'd meet a nice chap 'at the party'. It was all a bit weird really. Like going through the motions of life, how it was 'meant to be lived', when someone has already turned out all the lights and you are surviving in a post-apocalyptic world of empty streets and rubbish.

H was somewhere between awake and asleep, the chemo was kicking in and, although he hadn't been sick, largely due to the very powerful anti-sickness drugs, he was clearly being knocked sideways. Pops was tired but pleased to be with us.

I told them both about the 'Blue Moon' and Pops was quite interested, so we went outside to have a look. It was framed within the iconic 'lollipop' circles at the front of the hospital. The coloured circles so distinctive in every public image of the building, the structure you couldn't miss as you drive through Bristol City Centre.

It was a bit magical - the shining moon that is, not the structures, the sight of which I still loathe. I couldn't help but wonder how amazing the moon's light would be, shining over Dartmoor, its secret nooks and crannies shaded by the silvery glow of a thousand 'Blue Moons' going back to ancient times, when life was short and seasonal and silent killers stole people away in the night. Cheery thoughts for the season...

I draped my scarf over Pops' tiny shoulders, it was chilly. She looked so small. We looked up into the night sky, momentarily entranced.

'I'm giving all my wishes to H,' I said.

Pops looked up. 'I just want to go home mummy' she said.

'I know luvvy, I know. And we will. As soon as H is better. We'll be home before your birthday.'

Was that a lie? Or a wish? I didn't know either way. Be positive, said beautiful Moon Goddess shining down, communing with my own Inner Entity. They were both right and I knew it. Never underestimate the power of positive thought.

Looking up to the sky underlined just how small we all are, each of us less than a tiny dot in the gloriousness of existence. Our lives seem so huge to us, so all important and vital. Individually we are nothing. Life is cheap in so many parts of the world.

Here we were going through a tsunami of suffering yet we were tiny, insignificant, and unimportant.

Yet for all our smallness we had this huge hospital working 24-7 to get H better, working so hard to get us home and back to an ordinary life, to our small Devon cottage, the cats, the chickens, Gardeners' World on a Friday night.

There was a nurse on the ward, all she wanted was another baby. When I told her about the 'Blue Moon' she got so excited. I suspected I knew what some of the other nurses were wishing for as well. I knew which one was out drinking cider, which one was hoping to surprise her husband at the end of the shift and that one of them was not partying but saving for a Transatlantic trip. So much world, so many lives, so much living.

Humbled and cold Pops and I caught the lift back to Ward 34, through the thought-bending double doors, past the giant twinkling Christmas tree.

'Come on Pops, I'll race you to the chocolate. Then it's a taxi back to Charly's House,' I said.

H was asleep. I opened the Cava and poured some into plastic cups from the water dispenser by the nurse's station. We wandered off to find the 'buffet of biscuits, crisps and chocolate' set up in the playroom.

A couple from Ward 35, whose daughter had been in and out of the ward for years – yes, YEARS – chatted to me for a bit. They had a quiet resignation about them, their chain store clothes telling of a chain store kind of life, not telling of a teenage daughter with a degenerative cancer which would render her totally dependent before she died, which she would, way before her time. Having marked the occasion with one child, they were rushing home to be with their other.

Humbled by the magnitude of the 'Blue Moon' I now felt something different again. Was it hope? Hope that at least if the docs could nuke out H's crazy blood, get him back on track, he would have a life again – we would all have a life again. But in giving me hope it underlined the very real possibility it could go either way. What exactly would 2010 bring? Life or death? That's what it came down to.

What didn't come, though, was the taxi. Pops and I waited in the huge person-less hospital foyer until 1am. Despite two phone calls assuring me a taxi was on the way; nothing.

Well, quite frankly, this was where I could take control. Pops was shattered. I was putting her to bed on the ward. Hospital bureaucracy could stuff its paperwork wherever the 'Blue Moon' wouldn't shine.

We caught the lift back to H and, as my son stirred, I tucked Pops into my bed and sat on the institutional chair. I sat and sat, looking at both my children.

Maybe wishes do come true. Realising all I had actually wanted that night, all I had really wanted to kick off the New Year with, was to see both my 'babies' sleeping under the same roof. I found myself smiling through the tears. Who knows how long I sat there before realising I was really cold and, actually, really rather tired.

Sticking two fingers up at the bureaucrats I rifled around in the laundry cupboard and grabbed two clean crisp sheets (a much better service than back home) and some hospital standard issue blankets. The bed next to H's suddenly looked very inviting. If there was an emergency admission during the night, I'd have to move.

For a few wonderful minutes I felt I had actually done something for the three of us. We three were under one roof. We three would wake up together on the first day of a fresh, shiny New Year. Even though it was breaking all the rules. Not a single person challenged me.

New Year resolution: Break More Rules.

Inner Goddess was back – and boy did she need to be.

CHAPTER FORTY-TWO

New Year's Day was spent on Ward 34. H was hitting the point where he didn't want to even try getting out of bed. He was dripped up to the hilt. Mum and dad arrived around lunchtime.

'Well, it gives me a day off cooking', said mum as we contemplated the big treat laid on by the hospital for January 1.

The day before we had all been asked what we would like for lunch – yes, the bureaucrats were allowing mere relatives the opportunity to have a two-course hospital meal. To celebrate the New Year. We had even been allowed to choose what we wanted off the menu the day before. It was a very generous offer considering the 'rules' refused to allow anyone else a meal in hospital. No, I'm not being sarcastic. Alright, rumbled.

I knew I was being critical of the 'regime' we were living under. I was aware I was being ungrateful despite NHS staff doing everything they possibly could to save my son. But my favourite word has always been 'why?' and gratitude would not change that. The word '*why*?' has the power to change the world. *Why* serve rubbish food in hospital? Jamie Oliver asked *why* they do in schools, and look what happened there!

The 'Grumpy Old Woman' inside me really didn't think a two-course hospital meal was much of a treat. Couple of courses in The Ivy, Michael Caines' Gidleigh Park, cup of tea at The Savoy... Maybe I'm just hard to please. Or maybe it was just that hospital food was utter crap.

I tried not to dampen Mum's excitement. As gestures go it was pretty poor, the food was not exactly up to much. Alright. It was crap.

So many people said before Christmas 'oh yes, Christmas is actually great fun in hospital. There's loads of presents and visitors and a really good atmosphere.'

Well, we'd managed to miss all that, having been shipped out just in time. For some reason I had expected New Year would be 'fun' too.

Drowned lasagne and a roast – of indeterminate meat – hardly hit the high notes, though I have to say my dad's face lit up at the bowl of apple pie and custard (or was it crumble?).

H ate nothing, Pops not much. I think we both knew she didn't want to have to go back to Charly's House, even to escape the moth-eaten tinsel dangling about here and there.

I made tea in the parents' kitchen. The ward was fairly empty, which was a good job really. The effort of actually having to smile and make conversation was just too much by that point. Severe dose of *miserable cow* syndrome on my part.

After we had just sat, on the ward, doing nothing but keeping our upper lips stiff, I suggested mum and dad went back to Charly's House. There was no point in them staying. Dad didn't have a clue where he was anyway, and mum was hardly the life and soul, probably on account of her having run out of cheery conversation some years previously. Pops was agitated and tired. It was too much for all of us really. H and I could watch a film, do some sewing. Pops could have an early night.

By the time the three of them had left, H was shattered. And I was mentally seeking out ways of lengthening the rope leading to the end of my tether. How many more months of this? Three, four, five? Oh my Goddess. Time to find a shop selling very long ropes. No, not for that – but I did need some slack.

Solace was to come in an unexpected guise, one that took me completely by surprise. (No, not a fireman, though I wouldn't have said no...). But before then there was something I had to do. Something I had been putting off for far too long. The dreaded DLA forms.

Disability Living Allowance is a Government benefit which was, at the time, paid for people who are ill. The illness itself is means tested. If you are not very ill but a bit ill you qualify for the bottom rung. If you are fairly ill and incapacitated then you are entitled to the middle amount. And if you are very seriously ill then you qualify for the highest amount. And you do not have to be working to get it, which meant H qualified for DLA, at the highest amount because he was, like all the others on the ward, very seriously ill.

It's a peculiar and distressing process. To ensure you are not scamming you have to fill out a hideous form asking questions like:

'Tell us about the help or encouragement the child needs with medical equipment'.

Or: 'Tell us roughly how many times a day the child needs help'.

And: 'How many nights a week does the child need help?'.

He's living in a bloody high dependency oncology ward with numerous highly-trained staff!

The form took so much time to disseminate there was even a process you could go through if it's thought the applicant was likely to die before the process was completed. I found the form distressing, as did many others I spoke to. All the doctors and social workers and DLA officials already knew H would qualify for the highest level, before I'd dotted a single 'i' on the form.

Certain illnesses qualify, full stop. And you can't scam H's diagnosis. He now came complete with a sheaf of paperwork so extensive we'd soon need a small pack donkey to carry it around with us. So why, I lamented to anyone who would listen, why could two accredited consultants not sign a simple form confirming the qualification? A simple solution to a hideous scenario. It would save so many people hours back at DLA HQ. Indeed, you could probably fund a small principality off the back of the savings. Or pay a few dozen more nurses.

'*Oh no Madam, that's far too sensible*,' said the man in the *Ideas Office* located somewhere at the bottom of the rainbow's pot of gold.

'We can't have a simple system in place. It would confuse far too many people who are busy plodding away at the coal face of paperwork. And Madam, may I point out it would make far too many computer experts redundant. They need to be building complex systems to make life easier. Yes, I know these systems aren't able to talk to each other Madam, we do know that. But it does make life so much more interesting, don't you think? It would be far too sensible if we had one system and everyone knew what was happening and it would make life far too simple for those of you out there applying for these things. Besides, it will take you several hours Madam, to fill these forms out. We are actually helping you out here Madam, by giving you something to do. Thank you and Good Day to you', said the man from the *Ideas Office*, as the wooden hatch slammed onto the grimy wooden counter, missing my fingers by inches, shutting out reality.

At one point I had said to our CLIC Sargent social worker Lin I wouldn't bother with the DLA forms. It appeared that response was a common scenario and she persuaded me to carry on with them – they had even written a crib sheet to help respond to some of the questions, because so many parents found the forms difficult.

Some of the questions were so ridiculous it was hard not to feel you were existing in a parallel universe. Actually we were, but we all had to continue labouring under the common illusion we were, in actual fact, part of the real world.

When I discovered what we were in line for, I was stunned. My earnings had plummeted but I had enough to keep paying the bills in Devon, hang on to our home, keep body and soul together in Bristol. But the extra each month meant I'd not have to watch every single penny. It also meant something else – apart from extra stuff for H and Pops it meant I could go out and buy myself some clothes. Hell, I needed some new clothes, new or otherwise.

It was a relief to think there would be some extra coming in. Hospital living was expensive, having no kitchen was expensive, buying H and Pops little extras was expensive. It was balancing out a bit. Not putting petrol in the car, knowing my bills were considerably lower (well, not the water rates, South West Water were still charging me top whack even though the house was empty and the water turned off) because we weren't living in the house. But I was buying meals out – and not just for us. I was also having to fill two fridges – one in hospital to encourage H to eat whatever whenever. The other back at wherever our 'base' was at the time.

Friends and home town charities had been incredibly kind. Stuff arrived, cheques and notes and vouchers were posted. I had been given a couple of small grants via CLIC Lin. Money was tight. What am I saying? I still worried incessantly about money. Money cost me sleep. Now the cost of cancer had to be factored in as well.

At least I knew I could pay Magda because of the generosity of remarkably caring friends and a couple from mum and dad's

Dorset church. No grants. No loans. No re-mortgaging. I wonder how much straight jackets DO cost?

I had to sort out the ghastly DLA forms first. At least the man from the *Ideas Office* was right about one thing – it gave me something to do.

H slept. Pops cried herself to sleep. I filled out the forms.

CHAPTER FORTY-THREE

New routines emerged as the days went by. I'd regain consciousness around 6am as H's vitals were checked then doze for a couple of hours, mind racing. I was always happy when H went back to sleep. He needed to sleep. Conserve his energies, which anyone could tell were ebbing day by day.

I'd sit up, wriggle into the night attire I'd thrown off during the night, hoping no rogue doctor or unexpected nurse pulled back the curtain during my bed gymnastics. I hate sleeping in anything though I wish it could have been Channel No 5, like Marilyn Monroe.

Grab toilet bag, towel, and clothes then walk to the shower, hoping it didn't squirt unpredictably and get my clothes all wet. For some reason the fact the shower leaked onto the main corridor gave me a ridiculous sense of satisfaction. *See*, said my 'Grumpy Old Woman' persona, *it's a real inconvenience having to use a public shower each morning, squirm past groups of health professionals who are all dressed up, shaved, made up, respectable while I'm just trying to be invisible, not feel so out of place and undressed in such a public space.*

I was also becoming increasingly aware my legs were getting

hairier and increasingly convinced I would merely be viewed by all the staff as 'the woman with hairy legs'. No one will have noticed. But clearly my sense of paranoia was increasing. In reality, it seemed I was becoming known as 'the woman with big boobs'. I still don't know how you walk across a busy hospital ward and down the corridor with big boobs, no bra without being noticed and wobble free. At least I could laugh about it with Tam and the housekeeper.

Anomaly number goodness knows what (no, not a rip in the space and time continuum); somehow, it's OK to walk across a campsite with your wash bag and towel in your nightie but it's not OK to do the same in a hospital ward. It makes you feel like even more of an outsider. Even more uncomfortable, out of place.

By the time I got back to H's bed he was awake, not wanting breakfast. I'd lift the end of my bed, leaving the bedding in and push it back up to meet the wall. Tidy around. Pull up the institutional chair, the dull turquoise colour a familiar annoyance.

A nurse would deliver some meds in syringes, for me to give H. I'd make myself a cup of *Redbush* tea (snigger if you want to), offer H toast he wouldn't eat, and see if he would drink some fruit juice.

We'd wait for Pops to arrive. In the post 'festive' hiatus there was no school so doctors' rounds punctuated the wait. Polite enquiries. Temperature fine. Any concerns? If it was one of 'our' doctors it was always more satisfying somehow. When it was a stranger or a little-known entity there didn't seem much point really. I'm not very good at 'polite' conversation, it always seems so pointless. As long as I knew H was doing OK, all was well.

Mum and dad went home, cousins Debbie and Terry arrived to look after Pops for five nights. The atmosphere lightened.

It was good to see Debbie again – back to proper coffee - and both H and Pops were pleased to have her back. No masks this time! I was so grateful to them both for coming to help, step into the breach. Magda was not due to arrive until the following week. I knew how hard it was for mum to look after dad and Pops, though I'm sure Pops did much of the 'looking after'. It had been hard for Dad to be away from home, it must have been draining for them all.

Debbie and Terry arrived, full of energy. And plenty of funky new cardigans. They enlivened Pops, we reminisced about the Italian adventure (Terry had hosted it in her and her husband's glorious villa), fussed over her and I knew she could relax a bit more in a way she couldn't with grandma.

One lunch time H was well enough to leave hospital, so all five of us trotted up to our pizza place and had a glorious meal. It was such a treat to be able to spend time with cousins rarely seen, be able to watch both my children being 'normal'. Having some fun. It was also still a delightful novelty to be 'having lunch out'. After years of full-time work – rarely a lunch break – followed by years bringing up children when there was barely time to pee let alone eat around lunch time, well, lunch out. Just glorious! And no washing up.

We managed to get a large round table not too close to anyone else. It meant I could relax a bit, hoping no one would sneeze on H, pass on something nasty like chicken pox or measles. We took pictures, we laughed, we talked about family, drank wine. Terry wouldn't let me the pay the bill and it was really good not to feel so responsible, for a brief moment, for absolutely everything.

Debbie's husband, Nic, arrived after three nights to take her home, with their son Ollie. They all whisked Pops off to the docks and they went on The SS Great Britain, returned with torches for the children from the gift shop. It was easy to forget, trapped inside the ward, just what a cultured city Bristol was, a city oozing history (albeit some of it dodgy) and art and life. It almost felt like Pops had been on holiday. I was so chuffed she had had some fun.

While they had been out, I was in hospital with H. His haemoglobin levels had dropped so low he had to have a blood transfusion. However regular they were, however much a part of the treatment they became, I still hated the thought that someone else's blood was being pumped into my son's veins. Don't get me wrong. I was grateful H was being helped by complete strangers, complete strangers who would give their own bodily fluids to help someone they would never meet. (Memo to self – start giving blood again!).

But it was a double-edged gift. I couldn't get the fear out of my head. What if the blood hadn't been screened properly? What if the person who gave the blood didn't know they were HIV or had CJD or some other killing disease that would snuff out H's life further down the line? That one had already made global headlines; it wasn't an irrational fear. I was also sad that the blood H had been born with, the blood which had circulated around his innocent little body, was gradually being replaced by other people's because he was ill, because he had contracted such a horrible disease. It was yet another potent emotion mix – gratitude, intense and sincere. But fear my son was being pumped full of a 'killing cure' and alien blood.

As a mum you just have to swallow it, get on with. But it's hard to watch your child being pumped full of stuff, all the time hoping it will heal, not harm. The hour or so it took each time (was it longer? It felt like it) left me feeling tense. By the time H was unhooked my shoulders were hunched up around my ears and it felt like every sinew in my body was stretched out to impossible lengths. Were my thoughts rational? I may never know. Hope I never know.

One lot of blood H was hooked up to really freaked me out. Within minutes – and think me irrational, do, I thought I was at first – I was convinced he began to smell differently. My son began to smell of stale, overcooked vegetables (or was that just the waft coming from a food trolley?). As I called a nurse over, she wrinkled up her nose and then the alarm went off on the pump pumping the blood into H's wiggly. Lovely nurse restarted the pump but within minutes the alarm went off again. The smell was still there. My son had less than a third of the bag of blood but the doctor took him off it. It turned out the blood was not clotting right and kept blocking the tube. Within a few hours H smelt OK again but I was so relieved he had not been given the whole bag of blood.

During their stay Debbie and Terry performed a Herculean task. As H was now swine flu free – hurrah! – we had to vacate Charly's House. It was now time to move to CLIC House where we had been allocated a room with a double bed, a single bed and a sofa bed. My hard-working, resourceful cousins packed all our stuff up and moved it to CLIC House. They also cleaned the three-story town house which had been 'home' for the last month. And all without a car.

I do not know how we would have managed without them. We had been given so much stuff and we had acquired so much stuff and I had bought stuff – yes, a bit of vintage china, maybe a few books. My excuse was Christmas. People had been so generous! So kind! There were four cardboard boxes filled with chocolate and luxury biscuits alone. Boxes of Christmas presents, kitchen utensils, mugs, glasses, books, clothes, paperwork, more paperwork, books. Now it was all crammed into one room with a tiny shower squeezed into the corner.

When H was well enough to leave hospital for a few hours, we all trooped up to CLIC House so he and I could see our new 'home from home'. It was warm and welcoming, the faded elegance on the outside giving way to worn comfort on the inside. Funded by CLIC Sargent, supported by countless fund-raising efforts, the home had two managers who were very kind and always made time to help and listen.

The set up was simple. You were given a key to your room, shown the linen cupboard from which you could help yourself and left to your own devices. It was a communal house with plenty of bathrooms, toilets, random showers, a huge living room, a small one, a playroom (complete with pool table) a telephone you could dial landlines for free, a room just for teenagers, two kitchens and all over three floors. With a garden and a laundry room with commercial style tubs and a large tumble dryer. It was like an oasis. There was even parking for people who had cars with them. A real 'Holy Grail' in Bristol.

'Hello Sharon', said a woman I'd met on the ward, her daughter recently admitted with bone cancer. We chatted as cooking smells wafted out of a large kitchen. Pops and H went off exploring. She said they had only discovered the cancer when their daughter broke her arm and had been forced to move back to Devon from where they were living in Spain. They weren't just between homes, they were between countries.

'Wait until you see your room,' said Terry. Pops rushed on ahead, leading us up two flights of stairs. Debbie and Terry had carried everything up two flights of stairs! What could I say?

As we rounded a corner at the top of the grand stairs Room 9 came into view. Pops opened the door, she seemed excited. The room felt huge. It was clean, tidy and scattered with familiar things. But it was the view out of the windows which hit me. We were high up and the view across Bristol was awesome. It had been good from Charly's House, but it was even better from here. Almost opposite our room was a small kitchen, the 1970's Formica topped table in front of the window drew attention to another stunning view, overshadowing the cheap functionality which screamed 'everything here is donated'.

H was tired, so he curled up on the sofa in our room and he and Pops watched telly for a bit before he and I, reluctantly, went back to Ward 34, a Co-op green Thai curry from a plastic tray (fresh coriander? You're havin' a laugh), shortbread biscuits and however many episodes of Gavin and Stacey we could cram in before lights out.

CLIC House wasn't home. But it was the closet we had and it felt comfortable, its recycled vibe adding a layer of reassurance, familiarity and calm. At least we knew where we would be until we went home. I figured it was safe to think that. Surely?

The charity house certainly felt as if it was the gateway to a new phase in Bristol. Terry had to leave us the next day, her own life, business and husband pulling her back. Magda was not due to arrive until Sunday, so the hospital had graciously allowed Pops to stay on the ward with us on Saturday night. All three of us were looking forward to it and it took the edge off having to say goodbye to Terry.

Pops was reluctant to say Ciao to Terry. Almost as soon as my glamorous, designer clad cousin left Pops was in tears. Excited to be with us in hospital, sad to say goodbye to another carer – a night of films and popcorn promised. I felt she was becoming more bemused as each week went by.

I also knew she was nervous about Magda arriving. I couldn't tell her, but so was I. What if it didn't work? What if Magda couldn't get on with Pops? What if Pops didn't like Magda? This was a monumental undertaking for all three of us. I had not been able to CRB check Magda myself; it had all been done through personal recommendation and trust. Was I mad?

I had done all this on gut instinct. I had to trust my intuition. If this failed, I would be forced to leave H alone at night, however sick he got. I still had to find people to care for Pops Friday and Saturday nights as I could only pay Magda to look after Pops for five nights a week. It wasn't just about money. Seven days a week would be too intense for anyone, carer and the cared for. It was an unusual set up. It had to work.

I reasoned at least there would be structure for Pops. I looked over at my seven-year-old daughter, laying on the hospital bed next to H, his scalp pale, his face gaunt. They were both laughing at a cartoon. We had more than 24 hours together. It was a wonderful feeling. To enjoy it I had to block out the fears.

That night, watching both my children sleep, I called out to every benign entity in the universe, asking for H to get well and Pops to thrive. And please, please let everything work out with Magda. Inner Goddess responded with a curt *'well, it's a bit late now, isn't it'*, but I could tell she was smiling really. I would make it work with Magda. It would be tough on her too and the job description would have put most people off. I felt she had to be the right kind of person. I was gambling on her being just the right kind of person.

Meanwhile it was off to the hospital laundry room for clean white sheets. Don't get used to such regular clean sheets I told myself – well, there had to be some compensations to living in a hospital. Yes, LIVING in a hospital.

Day 56 in the Bristol Hospital Sanatorium – said with a broad Geordie accent in the style of Big Brother – and Sharon is trying on her straight jacket.

'Do you think my boobs look big in this?' said Sharon, wondering how on earth she was going to be able to undo the row of buckles at the back.

Until the fire alarm went off. 'Well officer,' said Sharon, 'what are you like with buckles?'

CHAPTER FORTY-FOUR

If I had to calculate the number of boxes of tissues I personally got through during our time in Bristol, it would be embarrassing. Most of them were sobbed into during the second round of chemotherapy. It was the most uneventful round, probably our calmest time in Bristol.

Magda was about to arrive. Neat, caring Magda her hair tied tight back from a pale face, the shadows under her eyes accentuating a seriousness which belied the fun beneath. Eat your heart out Nanny McPhee, Magda was Poland's answer to Mary Poppins in the trenches. Well, in my head she was.

One minute she was an unknown, the next it was as if she had always been there. Magda was serious in her look and her approach. Well organised, dedicated and calm. I was none of those by then, yet I'd become a boss. I was now the leader of a rag taggle bunch of four. No one knew what to make of us. We were still fairly unknown on the ward, because we'd been in isolation, virtually since arriving in the ambulance. It gave me an inordinate sense of satisfaction that people couldn't work out the dynamics. We had become the *Mad Hatter's Tea Party* of Ward 34. We defied all classification; we were an unusual group. Siblings tended to be sometime visitors and carer number two was invariably 'the partner'.

Magda's arrival gave me a dilemma. How do I be a *boss*? I had employed Magda to look after Pops five nights a week and we had agreed a salary, but we had not really agreed terms and conditions. How could you for such a scenario? We were all of us on a learning curve.

I figured the best way to kick everything off was retire to our favourite pizzeria for lunch. We had the all clear to take H out of hospital for a couple of hours, it was the logical thing to do.

Actually, there wasn't anywhere else we could go. I had not been able to prepare a lunch, going to CLIC House to have lunch meant me shooting off to buy food in a blind panic, having no idea what Magda liked and there wasn't anywhere in the hospital we could go and chill over a bite to eat.

Have I mentioned the inadequacies of the hospital canteen? It was certainly not drip friendly for H. It was tightly packed with a variety of chairs and high stools and was very public. Plus, there was the matter of my run in with a dreadful woman server who wanted to charge me double whack for a very inadequate Americano I tried to get an extra shot of Espresso into. Oh yes! The food was dire and overpriced. One decent strength coffee cost more than my daily food budget at home! There must be an art form to offering up unappetising sandwiches, rip off crisps and sausage rolls which looked more like cladding for pipes than food.

Indeed, this particular canteen should have been proudly displaying a certificate issued by the *Dire Food Standards Authority*, they would have breezed through to a five-star rating. It was also exploitation. Not just for minimum wage staff, but for patients and carers who needed sustenance the dire canteen and junk food machine dispensers were often the only option. It's not hard to make an effort with simple food at reasonable prices, enjoyed in pleasant surroundings. Staff smiling courses would have been a start. As these thoughts spilled out, I realised just how grumpy I was becoming.

Buck up, said Inner One.

Oh alright, said frustrated Grumpy Woman glaring back.

From what I remember, Magda parked her jeep near CLIC House and met us on the ward. She looked much as I remembered her from our brief meeting back in December, though maybe a bit more serious. Maybe she was nervous too?

It was all a bit awkward at first and after a bit of perfunctory chat, the sort of polite enquiries as to her journey, finding somewhere to park OK, not getting lost – the sort of thing I abhor – I dived straight in.

'How about lunch, our treat? Pizza OK?' I said.

'OK' said a cautious Magda, 'that would be good. Thank you.'

The sun was shining, we wrapped H up well and walked up the road, me gabbling like an idiot, pointing out various landmarks, giving a running commentary on places along the way. Pops was quiet, H too. I figured by the time lunch was over I'd have had to have proved to both my children, Magda was no longer a stranger, that she was now part of our very peculiar set up. I know, I know – it's an awful lot to ask of the humble pizza. I approached the restaurant scenario, as if we were at home entertaining. It was an unconscious ploy, but one I was getting used to.

Luckily a slightly more relaxed budget allowed these extravagances. We could never have lived like it at home. Those lunches, with great people who meandered through our life at the time, were the price paid for normality, a touching of base with the outside world, a place to go when all you had was a seat beside a hospital bed surrounded by drip stands, drug pumps, alarms and people. Endless, endless people.

Feeling like an Italian Mama (yay!) – complete with heaving cleavage and pasta complexion – I secured a table, bantered with the waitress, assured Magda she must have whatever she wanted and persuaded her, even though she was working, wine at lunch time was OK. I ordered a house red, Italian, of course. Would it bring us closer to the tumbledown village pizzeria, the one that existed in my head, like the ones we'd visited in Italy? Memo to self: travel more with my children!

Magda was great company and, with encouragement, even Pops began asking lots of questions about Poland, of her life in England. I was fascinated by the food she cooked, where she bought ingredients, the details of her own life.

Somehow everything felt better about the whole scenario – Magda was no longer a stranger to Pops, to H or to me.

'See' said smug Inner Goddess, *'told you it would be OK*!' And I knew it wasn't just the wine thinking.

I hoped the lunch helped Magda key into our scenario. We talked about the practicalities of how our set up would work. I said she must always be able to feel she could talk to me, that I knew this would be tricky and I appreciated just what a big ask her job was.

By the time H and I had to say goodbye to Pops that evening my daughter seemed a bit more relaxed. She held hands with Magda and I noticed Pops would talk directly to her, not look to me for approval. The pair of them had agreed a hair brushing regime, which was such a relief as Pops hated anyone but me doing it. She could still sit on her hair; it was so long.

As the pair of them walked out of the ward, chatting and holding hands, I could feel nothing but relief. I felt things may well begin to get a little bit easier. Pops would now feel she could have some control in our set up. I hoped the pair of them would get on well. I had, in effect, handed my daughter's welfare over to a stranger between sundown and school. But at least I no longer felt Magda was such a stranger.

'She's alright Magda, isn't she?' said H that evening.

'Yup H, I reckon you're right,' I said.

I sent silent prayers of thanks to my friend Jude, who had brought Magda into our life.

That night, whether out of relief or the continuing pressures of H's leukaemia, I cried. Hot silent tears of fear, relief, tiredness and frustration. Sewing helped, the crude folksy tree I started before Christmas now had a black cat on it, a basket of flowers and some bizarre red berries so out of scale and outlined in gold they should have looked odd and out of place yet, somehow, they fitted. Few more sequins ...

Funny, how even when you are out of place and don't fit, life takes on its own rhythms, becomes its own shape and designs its own space.

When the ward was quiet and H was asleep there was a calm like no other. And it was a calm I grasped. It told me we three WERE alive, we did have a life to go back to and I had to embrace exactly what we had in the here and now. You can be at the top of a mountain in a paediatric oncology ward, just as you can be down a pit on a Caribbean hammock.

I had known for years I should focus on what we had, not what we didn't.

'*Yeah*', said irritating Inner One '*been trying to tell you that for a few weeks now!*'.

CHAPTER
FORTY-FIVE

LIFE IS FULL OF RHYTHMS FROM YOUR HEART BEAT TO YOUR BREATHING, the music you listen to. I missed my music. And no crazy disco dancing, like at home, in here.

What do you mean you don't know what I'm talking about? You mean, you DON'T spontaneously get up and dance madly with your children. No, seriously! You don't? Oh crikey, you MUST. It's great fun. (Yes, just like Cher in Mermaids!).

H and Pops used to think I was barking mad – I know, hard to believe isn't it...? But once we agreed I wasn't allowed to behave like that in public, it was fine. They laugh, I laugh and the cats look on, utterly bemused. And trust me, when you're a working lone mum you gotta laugh as often as you can.

We may not have had our music to hand, but we did begin to develop new rhythms.

Pops and Magda would arrive just before nine in the morning and after huge hugs (while ignoring the big lump of non-porous mystery matter in my throat) I would walk her to school, which meant out of the ward and up the level five corridor where the hospital school was nestled between cleaning cupboards and secret storage spaces. Maybe we would chat with a teacher, talk about what Pops would do.

In the classroom seeing a bald child attached to drips galore with huge, Frankenstein scars ranging across a livid scalp, so pale they looked as if they had been living underground, lost the ability to shock us. The images had become dull recognitions.

Is that what soldiers see in war zones? Just a mass of blood and guts and body parts which merge into a horror so vivid it simply has to be ignored? The images on the ward, images of desperately sick children, had become familiar to us. But they weren't common place in real life. I knew people would be staring at us when we went out. H's pale bald head, a tube sticking out of his left nostril was as hard to ignore as his unnatural pallor. Hard not to stare.

In here, on Ward 34, you didn't have to force yourself not to look. You didn't, it had become 'normal'. It was our 'normal'. I think it's why, as time went on, I became increasingly frustrated by photographs on charity blurb showing cute kids with bald heads. Does it make people give more money? Or, as I suspected over time, did people avoid looking because it's too hard to see?

I suppose my frustration with the images was more about feeling helpless in our situation. My son was rapidly approaching total baldness – eyebrows and his beautiful long black eyelashes too - yet I didn't feel we were getting support. The one charity geared up to help us – CLIC Sargent – had many other families who needed help. And not enough resources or understanding from the world outside a hospital ward.

I knew it didn't mean our emotional or financial needs were any greater than those of any other family. But practically, our life was desperately challenging.

I had nobody to turn to for unconditional support. There was no partner to share this with, no one to hug me, hold me, no one who could say 'don't worry love, I'll sort that out'. I had no doubt there were plenty of people in the hospital who found me a right pain in the arse; my emotions were all over the place. I also knew not all partners are created equal ...

The walk back to the ward from the schoolroom was short. It was always a thoughtful journey.

Sometimes I would gaze longingly through the windows lining part of the corridor, the windows that looked out on to a tiny garden with a few pots and a bench, stones artfully placed all offering a small oasis in a world of airlessness. I never did understand the A4 photocopied sign taped to the door saying, 'No Entry'. The door was always locked. One day I even saw a fork and some gardening gloves, scattered soil on a slab and new plants planted. I wanted to stop and speak to the gardener, ask him or her if I could get permission to sometimes sit in their little area of loveliness. Except I never saw anyone there and anyone I asked knew nothing of the little garden.

How was that possible? A small, yet perfectly formed garden, no one knew anything about. Relief in a landscape of man-made materials so devoid of anything natural I had even begun to think the boiled carrots, plonked on plates, were as genetically modified as the drugs being pumped through H's stoic veins.

Talking of substances being pumped through veins... Magda and I loved decent coffee. We had fallen into a glorious weekday routine. Each morning we waited for doctors' rounds. When H was well – OK, I don't actually mean he was healthy, what with the leukaemia and all - I mean when he was doing 'well' on the remarkably unhealthy cocktail of drugs his weakened body was being forced to imbibe, all was 'well'.

Each week day morning doctors would do the usual, visiting each patient for an update. Updates were unremarkable. Discussions about the latest unplanned occurrence - such as an infection, another raised temperature, too much weight loss, antibiotic side effects, the need for stronger anti-fungal drugs, an urgent scan or X-ray, a rash, high levels, low levels, blood results, no blood results, platelets or a blood transfusion – were terrifying.

You may well think I was making too big a thing about this. But please bear in mind that what is a minor infection to you or me can mean life or death to someone with an immature, compromised immune system.

If you have a friend who is being treated for breast cancer, for example, you are encouraged not to visit if you have a cold. Hospitals ask you not to visit if you are suffering from diarrhoea or vomiting. There are good reasons. We already had the swine flu scenario under our belts. The implications for the hospital and other patients had been enormous. For young children who do not have fully developed immune systems, infections are particularly challenging. A minor infection can kill them.

When I was told not to let anyone get in a lift with H when he was neutropenic, (no immune system) in case they were infected with something so minor they didn't even know about it, I took it seriously. As seriously as I took doctors' rounds. Once doctors' rounds were over, we had a clearer idea of the shape the day was likely to take. Magda and I then waited for the teacher to arrive for H's morning lesson – if he was well enough – and we were free for almost an hour.

We headed for 'The Wild Wood' for our '*fix*', its black sign with curly white writing now as familiar as Ward 34.

The Wild Wood was a small, independent coffee shop almost opposite the hospital. If the green man (as in traffic light green man, not the wild man of the woods, though I was always on the lookout for him!) was with us, it took just a few minutes to get there.

With no apologies to my Devon coffee shop (who were by then second in the pecking order) The Wild Wood served up the best coffee I have ever had the pleasure to drink. And I am pretty fussy about my coffee, black – no sugar. Life is far too short to drink crappy instant.

Set up by a young Bristolian entrepreneur, whose aim was to serve up the best cup of coffee possible, this little gem did not just become a personal oasis, it actually changed the course of Magda's life...

Magda and I would order at the high wooden counter and plonk ourselves on opposite sofas at the back of the coffee bar café. It was not only sheer joy to sip top notch coffee, it was a delight to sit on a comfy sofa. Amongst the atmospheric, mainly music posters and many layers of paint holding the old building together, the pair of us chatted and plotted.

I found out more about Magda's life. I listened as the broken relationship which had, alongside the end of one contract and the possible start of another, given her a Pops/H-sized care slot in her work diary. I heard more about Poland and her family, life in Exeter, work. It also gave Magda the chance to know me a little more, for us to work out how we could make such a peculiar working relationship function.

The Wild Wood was like stepping into a shower which didn't cleanse but had the ability to caress back your own 'normal'. It gave me a chance to be 'me', not the stress cadet who related to everyone around her in a permanent state of turbo-charged angst. It was a chance to breathe. Never underestimate a good coffee in a good coffee shop; healing powers!

The more Magda and I talked, the more I realised what a gift she was in our life. Determined, highly focused and hard-working Magda was, if anything, far too hard on herself. I was astonished at just how quickly someone could take in our situation, align her own emotions so exquisitely to the scenario, and roll up her sleeves. She was also very good at doing Pops' hair, her long, long plait – cut only once since she was born – quite an undertaking.

We talked practical. We decided, each morning, over coffee

was the time to deal with the necessities of each day. I made it clear Magda must tell me if she had any problems with the set-up, and we had to work through it together. If ever there was a need to communicate openly and honestly with someone I barely knew, now was it.

After lunch, which the four of us would eat together on the ward by H's bed, Magda and I would take it in turns to have a couple of hours off. I would take Pops with me, to spend some time with her while Magda sat with H. Then Magda was free to wander as she pleased.

Pops' response was mixed. Chuffed to be with me, but not particularly thrilled at the prospect of 'not more shopping mummy'. But shop we had to, mostly for Pops because she was growing out of the few clothes we had with us. With dismay I realised Pops was growing in every direction, so the walk into Bristol city centre – with various hills – was good exercise for us both. And she needed clothes, which became increasingly hard to find. She was seven, but very tall for her age and I often had to feed Pops with whatever was available at the time. There was far too much fruit juice drunk – with its lashings of hidden sugar – and chocolate, crisps, sweets and biscuits on tap. What H wouldn't, or couldn't eat, Pops did. By the time she was out of children's sizes I was getting desperate to find new trousers for her. And tops that weren't covered in sequins (!) or inane, inappropriate logos like 'good girls just want fun' or 'Smile it's Saturday'. Some of the shopping trips were fraught. Pops hated trying on clothes. In my desperation to make those times count, make sure the time worked for Pops, we walked all over Bristol city centre and some of its hidden green spaces. By the time we got back to Ward 34 Pops would be sporting new trousers or a new top, but she would be tired and I would be exhausted, wrung out. But we had foodie places so there would be a nice cake, some juicy fruit, hopefully something decent for tea for Pops and Magda, a treat for H, yet another microwave ready meal for me.

While Magda was out, we three would usually watch a DVD, H propped up on pillows, Pops on my lap our arms wrapped around each other like we never wanted to let go.

When Magda got back maybe a cup of tea before saying goodbye to Pops, which became harder by the day.

I did talk to some of the other parents, a handful of whose faces I recognised from early on, glimpsed through the window in the door of Room 4. But increasingly I felt isolated, alone. I so often cried myself to sleep, my eyes were red and bug-like in the morning. I just couldn't face talking to people.

I also found I didn't want to be sociable with people, who were only on the ward overnight, or for very short periods of time. It was too hard to be friendly, polite, sociable. The effort it took was immense, and I was so fragile myself I couldn't be the me I am, the me who was chatty, open, comedic. I was becoming spikey, unapproachable and more frightened as every day passed.

The words 'forty per cent' haunted my waking and sleeping. I was terrified of the effect this nightly separation would have on Pops when we eventually got out of here – or worse. What kind of Mum would I be able to be to my seven-year-old daughter, if all three of us didn't make it home?

I felt, deep down, I was right to have Pops with us. But what if I was wrong? What if she was better off being in our home town, staying with friends, going to school, coming to Bristol at week-ends. But who would she stay with? Who would be able to bring her up each Friday? Take her back each Sunday. Where would she be allowed to sleep? Surely being parcelled around, being so far from us, would be worse for her than just being away from us during the night?

Permeating all of this was the reality of H's leukaemia.

Extreme weight loss, baldness, raised temperatures, vigilance for infection – seen and unseen.

I had never been so surrounded by people 24/7. Yet I had never felt so on my own. The pressure of knowing if I got this all wrong there would be repercussions, for years to come, became a pressure I had to try and shut out. Sewing helped enormously. Focusing on H's needs was essential. Being in the moment with Pops staved off some negative thoughts. But nothing seemed to stop the night crying which, I hoped, was as silent as it could be.

One night, just before the early hours vitals check, I was wiping away tears when one of the younger oncology nurses pulled back the curtains just a bit too quickly. I didn't have time to hide the pile of soggy tissues.

She smiled, checked H over and wrote the obligatory numbers on his chart before turning to me, concern etched over her face.

'Tell me what's wrong,' she said, the simple enquiry prompting more tears, her kindness just too much.

I burbled in hiccupped whispers. She listened. Here was a young woman with no offspring who had decided she would care for very sick, sometimes terminally ill children. She knew, as well as I did, she couldn't say anything that would make any difference to our situation. Yet somehow her quietness, her guts to even ask the question, was so humbling it helped give me a bit more to hold on to, a bit more to keep going through the second round of chemo.

It was just one example of how incredible H's nurses were. A handful had young children themselves but many of them were early in their nursing career yet they had understanding, an unexplained empathy, an innocence which afforded them the ability to actually care for their patients - and those of us consigned to the ward.

She made me a cup of tea, got me some more tissues. But more importantly she gave me something I have never quite been able to put my finger on. Maybe it was just that she had shared my experience, albeit from the outside in. Or perhaps it was simply that she was brave enough to work on the ward, to cope with what she saw, heard and mopped up.

I knew these nurses were not paid anything like their worth. It was a true vocation. The ward was frequently short staffed, and they didn't get much opportunity to drink tea or take a break. They often had to run between patients, so acute were the needs on this ward. I will always remain grateful for everything they did for H. And humbled by how they coped with the spikey malcontent I had become, riding a wave of fear, exhaustion and uncertainty.

At long last I was beginning to realise why so many patients' mums appeared on the ward with piles of cheap celebrity magazines and bottles of half-drunk coke. I hardly ever saw people reading books. There was no peace on the ward, I had even given up trying to read a newspaper let alone a book. Interruptions were near constant. I began to wonder what else was in the bottles of coke... now there's a thought.

Oh no lady, you're not doing that...

Why not? said a loud but naughty voice.

Because it's really not a very good idea, is it? came the swift reply.

And it wasn't.

But nor is putting cheese in a tube or jumping off a cliff attached to a long bit of elastic, is it?

CHAPTER FORTY-SIX

ONE OF THE THINGS I BEGAN TO TAKE GREAT COMFORT IN DURING THE second round of chemo, was plants. I found it hard to get my head round the idea my son's nine-year old body was being pumped full of so many rabidly toxic chemicals, when I had tried hard to be organic and steer clear of noxious chemicals in our home. I know, hilarious, isn't it!

One day I almost ended up in A&E because some of his wee squirted in my eye. Much frantic washing out with tubes of saline sorted it, but one red sore eye underlined how evil the chemo was. How can it heal? Look what it was doing to H.

I think it was Lovely Zoe who told me one of the chemo drugs H had already had was made from a chemical found naturally in a sea sponge. Others came from American May Blossom, another regime used extract from the bright blue periwinkle flower.

I wrote in the blog:

'Can you believe it? Some marine biologist, or an oceanologist, or a random diver must have delivered a sample to a scientist, somewhere, who did some research and some medical bod somewhere discovered a formula that has ended up treating AML. How on earth could such a

connection have been made? From sea bed living to chemotherapy in a thousand 'easy' steps. I mean, WOW! Amazing or what?! I have always known Mother Nature is utterly amazing... It is comforting to know such magic reached the depths of a cancer ward for children'.

As I wrote the blog, I noted we were sharing Ward 34 with a three-year old, two five-year olds, an eight-month old baby girl and two other babies. Seven children fighting cancer.

At the time I knew seven other people fighting cancer. Back in Reading a friend of mine was bringing up her two youngsters, alone, after their dad died of throat cancer.

All these natural cures waiting to be discovered. Apparently rain forests across the world contain sufficient diversity of life to find cures for all cancers – or did I dream that? So why are we raising them to the ground for commercial gain?

The final blog of January heralded fabulous news:

'The last few weeks have been gruelling mentally and physically, but barely four hours ago I received a phone call telling me H's latest bone marrow results (op on Tuesday just gone) show he is still in remission. It is great news. It is the best there is!!! It is all worth it!'

I also had to tell people '*H is still being utterly amazing! He has his moments (far shorter than mine or Pops') but he has shown a maturity, an emotional intelligence, an acceptance, some kind of understanding that continues to humble me. I have always said I learn from my children – daily!'*

The next round of chemo was due to be the most gruelling. Five days of 24/7 drugs set to make him very sick.

In the meantime, we had four days off. Magda's care and support continued to be remarkable, and though we would miss her I dispatched her back to Exeter so she could have a mini break from us. And H was off the yellow gunk, his liquid food.

Time to sleep, eat, cuddle my children and explore Bristol.

We had, in CLIC House, proper beds, a kitchen with a cooker, table, chairs, a clean fridge and, wonderfully, a garden. Never again will the simple pleasures we thought we already cherished ever be taken for granted.

If we could import Oscar Wilde and Ruby Tuesday, along with six ex bat chickens, we'd be in heaven.

CHAPTER FORTY-SEVEN

We were on the third round of chemo, back in the same bed 9, but a day behind schedule as the ward was closed down on Sunday, because of sickness and diarrhoea. Must have been serious as there's plenty of that around anyway.

H was weeing for Britain, which is quite normal with the chemo. We usually had at least four wee bottles by first thing, all of which have to be taken to the sluice room so all outputs can be measured. Except the ward had run out of wee bottles, so all the children not in nappies had to pee into sick bowls. These, of course, have far more potential for accidents... which can be a challenge with such toxic effluent. Couldn't find the reel of plastic *biohazard tape*... Can't wait to get back to bare feet.

H was a bit fed up. He couldn't even watch a Dr Who DVD for a bit of escape because we couldn't find a telly that worked. I tried to rig up the laptop, but the wiring was too tricky and would have been a danger to our nurses.

You leave the ward for a few days and when you come back something mysterious has occurred; the working tellys have disappeared and Lord Lucan has nicked all the remotes. The playroom was closed because it – and all the toys – was being deep cleaned. We couldn't leave the ward because H was hooked up to chemo and his little mate Sam was in isolation, because of a sick bug. H had little to do but wander the ward, pushing his drip stand. Nothing I said or did helped.

Next thing he's locked himself in the toilet and refuses to come out. The SAS crack nurse squad plunged in, nurse Rachael opened the door from the outside, entered H's new realm and talked him down.

All he wanted, she reported back, was a bit of space. The ward was so noisy that morning. There was no filter on visitors, whatsoever. If the bed next door wanted to have four grandparents, two aunties, a cousin and what looked like half The *Adams Family* visiting, they could. And they did. It was ridiculous, and I told Jamie so. He didn't disagree but there was absolutely nothing he could do about it. We had to put up and shut up. The noise that morning had been so bad even H's hospital teacher, who was trying to give him a lesson on the ward, had given up early. When I tried to ask the mum in the family if they could be a bit quieter, I received, shall we say, a rather 'frosty' response, from the whole clan.

One of the other dads on the ward, a serving police officer, made a poignant observation. 'Well,' he said, as he was sorting out his son's feeding tube, 'class is no barrier to illness.'

They were a lovely family from Cornwall; he was full of common sense and quiet dignity. Their three-year-old son had a brain tumour, they had been in the loop several months. Mum was caring for their two other children, one a baby, at CLIC House. It was the family we had seen round the Christmas tree when we went for a walk, just before the New Year. Their hopes were pinned on a pioneering treatment offered at Great Ormond Street Hospital, London. To get there, dad had to take his son on a train. The fares were very expensive. I never heard them complain.

It transpired all H wanted was to watch a film so he could shut out all the noise. He was so fed up and the chemo was already beginning to make him feel rubbish.

We got special permission, from his consultant, to leave the ward for three quarters of an hour. A short walk to the crystal shop and a lemonade in The Wild Wood helped. In that time magic happened. Daffodil Yellow Housekeeper found him a new TV so, after almost two days without. H can at last watch some DVDS, of which we had a growing collection.

The blog read:

'Feel strangely proud of my son's act of rebellion, for which I should have been very cross with him. But his protest – which I now know he thought through very thoroughly before ending up in floods of tears asking for his Mum – actually created a pathway of understanding with several people who I feel often don't really see H, because he just gets on with it in a way not all the patients do'.

After H's drama I returned to the ward, with Pops, following a successful food foraging expedition, and walked slap bang into *Narnia*. A beautiful, blonde 'hippy chick' was playing the harp. Yup, a huge harp stood in the middle of the ward. Such beauty in such a challenging environment was simply too much and, yes, I burst into tears. It was breath-taking. Glorious!

I persuaded the harpist to play outside the door of Room 3, so Tam and Sam could hear her properly. Despite mercilessly taking the piss out of my fist of damp hankies – in sign language through the narrow window in the door - it put a smile on their faces too. Maybe we really were in *Narnia,* just without the heavy fur coats...

The harpist had been organised by the hospital school, which was staffed by some remarkable teachers, they 'got' the needs of so many children on the ward.

When H was well enough he – and I – were enchanted by the story tellers who regularly roamed the wards. In a clinical world of high-tech healing to have small slots of random enchantments, in the form a fairy tale re-told, was wonderful in a mystical full-of-wonder- way. It was how we had discovered the Eastern European hag Bab Yaga, who lived in a hut on running chicken legs and had a fence made of skulls from her victims. Magda knew the witch from her childhood. Well, not personally, through books, obviously. H adored witches and when he wasn't reading stories about them, he was drawing cauldrons.

CHAPTER
FORTY-EIGHT

HOSPITALS ARE BUILT TO HEAL PEOPLE, YET THEY ARE NOT NECESSARILY places of healing.

In the early hours of Sunday morning H was fast asleep and, as the ward was empty – a first! – we were both making the best of it. Suddenly all the lights went on. Peering at us through the brightness was a woman doctor I'd never seen before. And a 'bank' nurse who had travelled from Cardiff, to do a shift. I didn't know her either.

I heard the doctor say to H

'How's the rash, is it itching at all?'

Fortunately for the pair my brain was a bit slow, having just been woken up.

I sat up, blinking in the glare.

How on earth was H meant to answer a question like that? Of course he wasn't sodding well itching, he'd been fast asleep. It doesn't take seven years medical training to figure that one out, surely? He rolled over, silently, and huddled back into his quilt, which he preferred to scratchy blankets.

Both women scuttled off, my withering, silent glare poisonous enough to grace a Shakespearian stage, I felt sure. Un-bloody-believable. I got up, stomped across the ward and turned the lights off, got back into bed.

It wasn't a dream. H's medical notes confirmed the intrusion. Much of the previous week, while H had been hooked up to chemo 24 hours a day, the ward had been horribly noisy and unsettling. When all he'd wanted to do was sleep, the rest of the ward seemed to be partying.

It's a tough scenario. Very sick children and their families having a good time versus a very sick child wanting peace and sleep. There is no middle ground.

In 'be-careful-what-you-wish-for' part two, later that day we moved into Room 3. H had 'loose stools', which the doctors felt was not drug related. We were in our 'own' room again, encircled by four walls, protected from noise.

The euphoria was short lived. No access to the parent's kitchen, no sluice room ambles, no access to drinking water. More importantly, what had prompted H's diarrhoea? Samples were taken.

I knew H wasn't doing great. Mum had managed a trip to Bristol that weekend, by herself on the train. My brother had gone to Dorset to look after dad. It was a break for mum, and a chance for Pops to have some grandma time.

It had not been a successful weekend for anyone.

My brother had been delayed on Friday night, traffic or work; it was always one or the other. It meant mum was constantly worrying about dad. My brother had to leave early, because he had important stuff to do, so the lunch we had managed to spring H for was rushed because mum had to get home earlier than planned. As it happened H projectile vomited all over the restaurant table. The Wagamama staff were very understanding.

Soon after I had moved all our things from the ward, into Room 3, the phone rang. Dad was in intensive care at Salisbury District Hospital.

Mum told me he had pneumonia. He was on a ventilator because he couldn't breathe unaided.

'I thought he wasn't right when I got home yesterday,' said mum. 'It was like he was hallucinating, he kept talking utter nonsense. Nothing made sense. Neil said he'd been really odd all weekend.'

'What did the doctor say?' I said.

'Oh, I didn't call the doctor about it. I thought he'd probably be OK in the morning. I managed to get him to bed. I hardly slept though. He kept waking up and rocking about, as if he was on a boat.'

True to her 'I-didn't-want-to-make-a-fuss' roots, mum had not called a doctor until gone six o'clock Monday morning. Within minutes an ambulance was on the doorstep. Dad was now on life support and in a drug induced coma. His brain had apparently been starved of oxygen, aggravating the vascular dementia.

As I was sat on my favourite (not) turquoise institutional chair, head in hands, the phone rang again.

'Hello, how are you all doing?' It was other grandma. 'Thought I'd better let you know. Ron's in hospital. They admitted him this morning. They're not sure what's wrong.'

Two granddads; one in a Salisbury Hospital, one in a Plymouth Hospital.

No time to dwell on it, grab a bedpan. No ... oops, too late.

'Sorry H, I wasn't quite quick enough, was I? Shall we get some clean sheets? Here you are love, let's clean you up.'

I sat H on the chair, wrapped in blankets, while I stripped the bed and put on clean bedding, taken from the stash I had secreted during the move from ward to room. I made a mental note to let the nurses know the bed pan was not representative of the full ablution, for monitoring purposes. I was meticulous in cleaning the surgical mattress with wipes formulated for the purpose. Even cleaning products in hospital have a pecking order.

I spent the next few hours tracking down dad's consultant, between soiled bed pans. I had chats with a number of doctors in Salisbury, and, due to current circumstances, may even have sounded quite knowledgeable about hospital conventions. Funny that.

Although I was becoming increasingly concerned about H's condition, I was grateful we were back in isolation. It had enabled me to have some very heavy-duty conversations with hospital staff at Salisbury, in private. Mum was in shock. I felt as if I was her conduit, channelling information her way. It wasn't the first time in my life I thanked my profession of journalism. Asking questions, gleaning information, is an undervalued skill and besides, it made me feel I was doing something for my dad.

The blog degenerated into a burble;

'Silent screams can't be heard. When I have re-scraped myself off the floor it's onwards and upwards.

'It is the early hours of the morning. It is early hours with dad. Can only hope the doctors in Salisbury ... are as good as the doctors here in Bristol... All I need now is a magic carpet. And a jumbo-sized packet of sanity. Anyone know where I can get one? Yeah yeah, I know, from the marble shop. Memo to self: 'Magic carpet to marble store to restock, supplies diminishing rapidly.

Love to you all out there, Crazy Blood Mum xxx'

The blog dried up soon after that. I couldn't find enough ways to be cheerful in print. Inner Goddess remained silent.

CHAPTER FORTY-NINE

Walking back from the schoolroom, after dropping Pops at school, I bumped into the head of nursing. I liked Hazel. We'd first met at the high-level meeting – well, it was held on the top floor – soon after we landed in Bristol.

My first impressions of the compact matron of matrons had been of a woman who was efficient, hard-working and with a tough outer veneer she knew when to toss aside. The Hazel I bumped into that day had dropped the no nonsense façade and her enquiry was heartfelt.

'I was sorry to hear about your dad,' she said, talking to me as an equal, not some random patient's mum. Had I made that much of an impression, or was I simply known within the management team as that *right pain in the arse*? I'd like to think it was the former. Her kind enquiry was much appreciated.

It seemed like word had gone around the hospital; she wasn't the only person to ask about dad in the coming days. Despite my views about NHS bureaucracy, I only experienced professionalism and caring from most of the individuals we met inside the hospital.

By the time I'd returned to Room 3, I'd made my mind up;

Pops and I were going to visit dad in Salisbury. It was just a question of working out when, and how.

There will most likely have been a conversation with Jamie, asking him if he felt I could leave H for a few hours. It was decided the best time to go would be the following day, Wednesday afternoon.

Armed with a Family Railcard, Pops and I set off with some scribbled train times and a vague plan. It had to be a bus to Bristol Temple Meads, a train to Salisbury followed by a taxi from the station to the hospital as it was too far out of the city centre to walk.

I couldn't help wondering if it was the last time I would see my dad. I felt his doctors had been open with me; I had asked very direct questions. The pneumonia, of indeterminate origin, they were fighting with drugs. But keeping his vital organs going was harder. If his liver, kidneys or heart failed, decisions would have to be made. There was also a question mark hanging over his state of mind, given the unfolding history. They confirmed probable vascular dementia.

One of the doctors also told me they suspected he had suffered, in the recent past, a series of mini strokes, which had most likely further diminished his brain function. There was also a suggestion being on life support itself, in the state he was in, could exacerbate a further deterioration of his mind.

'We have to look at his quality of life,' said one of the consultants, 'how was he before this happened?'

There's a question! My view was going to be significantly different from my mother's. Mum was due to meet us at the hospital later. I knew she was in a terrible state. We had a couple of our favourite M&S ready meals in a bag for her.

The tone of the ensuing conversation with the intensive care doctor, all on the phone before we set off for Salisbury, had been the suggestion that life support should be turned off, if the doctors could not see their way to dad regaining at least the same quality of life he'd had previous to the pneumonia. It was for the family to decide, said the consultant I spoke to, if they could get him through the pneumonia.

I tried to be upbeat about the journey, for Pops' sake. Apart from being draped in a boa constrictor – organised by the Bristol Hospital school teachers recently – a train ride was the most risqué thing we'd done since leaving Devon. Was it odd to feel a sense of freedom, even though we were only between hospitals? But it was also like an out-of-body experience.

I noticed, at Salisbury train station, a window box. It was planted with daffodil bulbs which were poking through, greeting the frosty air in their own bid for freedom, shaking off the shackles of an extraordinarily icy, snow-ridden winter.

Like the daffodils, I had to push through.

CHAPTER FIFTY

Pops and I arrived at the hospital before Mum, were shown to a waiting room set up for visitors. It was a cross between the parents' kitchen on Ward 34 – with a kitchenette comprising sink, toaster, microwave and drink making facilities - and the tiny 'family room' on the corridor leading to our ward. I noted the sofas were significantly cleaner. It was a large, bright room. The 'family' room for Ward 34 was tiny and had no window, just the narrow, metal wired opening in the door.

A nurse came in. 'Are you here for Mr Cook?' she said.

I nodded and she offered to take us through. Pops was glued to my side. I decided to go in to the ward. Mum was on her way but we had such a tight window, if she was late, I didn't want to risk losing the chance of seeing my dad.

We were led through intensive care to a bed on the far wall, in the right-hand corner. Pops held my hand. She'd had a crash course in bedside manners. I reasoned she could cope with this. I may have been wrong, but she would never have stayed on her own in the family room anyway.

There was no denying dad was a shocking sight. Drip stands, syringe drivers – one for morphine - a big pipe stuck in his mouth, attached to a pump, a catheter bag hanging, nutrition pump, an oxygen clip on his left index finger. The set up made H's scenario look tame. Oh God please don't let H end up in PICU (Paediatric Intensive Care Unit).

Pops stared. I held back tears (yes, I know, tedious!) moved forwards, touched dad's hand, stroked his arm, the skin a clichéd paper thin, wrinkled, grey with deep purple bruises pooling around his cannula. Vaseline was smeared round his mouth, stubble on his face. We stood for a while, my daughter and I. A nurse was checking levels, pressures, tubes, numbers, writing things on a chart. I don't remember what she looked like. I just felt a sense of respect. Despite the shock of it all, the place offered a sense of calmness and dignity. A sterile cathedral for the dying. Where on earth had that come from?

I said we would have to go, meet my mum, was it OK if we came back shortly?

'Just buzz your way back in and tell us who you've come to see. It's no problem,' she said. I arranged for a doctor to meet us in the 'family' room when we came back.

We'd just got to the canteen when mum walked in, with her friend Gwenda, one of the kindest, calmest people I've ever met. There is no etiquette for situations such as these. Mum looked drawn and fragile, her customary brown pink lipstick in place. I think she really appreciated the food parcel, admitted she hadn't eaten much since dad was driven away in the ambulance.

I was glad we'd arrived before mum. It meant I could walk her there and hold her hand when confronted with the reality of dad's condition. This was her first visit, though I had to bite my tongue not to ask why she had left it more than two days before coming, I figured she'd had more than enough on her mind. Besides, Dad would have had no idea she was there. Maybe the hospital had said not to come. In the beginning they had to restrain him, tie him down, his violent thrashings most likely a result of being starved of oxygen. Gwenda took Pops off for a walk while mum and I went back to dad's bedside.

The same kind nurse was there, took dad's personal toiletries from mum. I thought I saw she'd packed his aftershave. It was kneejerk stuff really. What does a man on life support want with aftershave? It was heart breaking. Mum was in a terrible state.

We stood by the bed for a while – oh for a turquoise chair - this time Mum holding his hand. I had to tell her I'd arranged for us to chat with one of the doctors, gently reminded her Pops and I had to leave soon, because I'd booked a taxi to get us back to the station.

'How is H?' she said, through tears.

'He's good Mum,' I lied.

I made us both a cup of tea. We sat and waited for the doctor.

'You know this isn't good, don't you mum?' I said, testing the water. She seemed to be holding it together. 'Do you understand what the doctors are saying?'

We both got out tissues. Mum handed me some photocopied sheets about vascular dementia.

'I thought you might find these helpful,' she said, handing them to me. I didn't have the heart to point out the situation had moved so much further on. Maybe this doctor could help her to understand, I didn't want to be the person who told her if Dad did make it through the pneumonia, we needed to consider turning off his life support. There is a reason why they call pneumonia *'old man's friend'*, even though my Dad was only 71 years old.

The conversation was just as hideous as I had expected it would be. When he arrived, the doctor reiterated what I had already been told, but I knew mum wasn't taking in the implications.

'I just want to have one more conversation with him' she kept repeating. 'I'm not ready to let him go.'

I looked at the doctor, we exchanged non-verbals. He assured us we could call the ward any time we needed to.

'Mum, do you understand what he was saying?' I had to ask, after he'd left.

Angrily, she looked at me.

'I'm a Christian Sharon. This is not a decision for me to make. It's down to God.' And that, as they say, was that.

I wished my brother could have been there, but he couldn't get time off work. He's self- employed. He made it in the following week.

As mum and I walked back to the canteen I was overwhelmed with the urge to get back to H. Where's David Tennant when you need him? Tardis!

Pops and I caught a taxi instead, hugging mum goodbye, promising to call her later, when we got back to Bristol.

As the taxi dropped us at Salisbury train station, I searched out the window box of sprouting daffodils. I missed growing things. I missed my garden, pots of herbs on our window sills, seeds finding their way. Even flowers in vases are now banned in hospital wards.

I knew I was going to miss my dad. Whatever news the next few days brought, he was already gone. If only I'd known how precious our last few encounters were going to become: a day by the beach in Sidmouth last autumn, talking on the phone about the lap top, falling asleep on a chair in Room 4, a roast chicken dinner at Charly's House, pouring him wine, the smell of his aftershave.

I had to leave my dad, so I could get back to my son.

CHAPTER FIFTY-ONE

After Dad's admission to hospital, events flurried thicker and faster than all the record-breaking snow we'd experienced over Christmas and New Year.

Amongst the phone calls, visits, diary crisis and chemo side effects, Pops and I managed another 'mercy dash' to Salisbury the following week. Dad's condition hadn't changed.

At some point during that time - I think the horror of it all blanked out the exact course of events – H was diagnosed with norovirus. The 'loose stools' – not so much loose as liquefied – had tested positive for the nasty little bug which caused raised temperatures, headaches, stomach cramps, aching limbs and effluent to gush out of both ends.

While it is virulent, norovirus is not particularly dangerous, though it is hard on the young and elderly, or, of course, those with compromised immune systems. Fortunately for everyone else doctors had already taken the precaution of keeping us in isolation. Were there others? For H it could have had devastating consequences. His bum got very sore and red and there were concerns it could get infected. He was well into the third round of chemo so his body was already waving a white flag.

There was only one place H could have caught the virus: On Ward 34. I was incandescent. Had I been right to feel uncomfortable about the needle I'd dropped in round two, found by the bed at the start of round three? I was furious that a 'deep cleaning regime' – it had been done twice – could have failed so spectacularly. Splashing around a few chemicals and wafting round a steam cleaner clearly wasn't working. This is hardly news. The likes of antibiotic resistant MRSA strains are killing people in our hospitals. But norovirus, on a high dependency paediatric ward, well, it's beyond outrageous.

Hadn't H been through enough already, I railed silently?

'We know' said Inner Goddess, sounding weary. *'Stop moaning and just get him through it.'*

I hoped I could help prevent an infection on his bum – I resorted to olive oil as a barrier, especially when the suggestion of a visit from a skin specialist who used a honey-based treatment never materialised.

I had learnt early on in H's treatment that the doctors, consultants and specialists would not discuss even the idea of alternative therapies or holistic treatments. I was not suggesting I fly in a Shaman from Papua New Guinea or smear my son with pungent unguents and bathe him in sage smoke. Now there's an idea that would cause a bigger sensation than the harp! But I did wish conventional medicine was more open to exploring the possibilities of plants. I do realise the research would be costly and raw plant material is variable. But when so much of conventional medicine is already based in pant lore – let's just mention sea sponge, American May Blossom and Periwinkle shall we! – *why* are minds not more open?

The idea of cleaning a hospital ward with little more than vinegar, lemon juice and bicarbonate of soda, maybe some lavender and tea tree oils, is probably not very appealing to the companies which make millions out of cleaning products. Yet if it works in the domestic arena, *why* aren't we trialling it in hospitals? Can it really be less effective than what's being used? It would certainly smell better. And be kinder to our beautiful but beleaguered earth.

Off my soap box. Back to H's plight. He'd stopped eating some days ago, so we were back to the yellow gunk. What made it so awful this time round was his being sick so often. The thin plastic tube leading straight to his stomach was prone to pop out when he was violently sick, which meant it had to be put back in again. He was getting more distressed each time it happened.

I found the look on his face distressing when he could feel it coming out as he was being sick. I kept thinking he was going to choke on vomit. We reached the stage when he would only let certain people put it back in. I think Jamie was one of them – or was it Chemical Ken - my mind was getting frazzled.

I had to climb on to H's bed, hold him in my arms as he was between my legs and talk to him all the while clasping him to me, trying to calm him down. I felt like I was facilitating the torture of my son as the tube was inserted. But I knew if we didn't get the tube in, he wouldn't get the nutrition he needed, which would make it harder for him to fight both the side effects of the chemo, and the norovirus.

The doctors were remarkable: Constantly monitoring every aspect of H's body. He had bloods at least once a day, via his wiggly, checking not just all the levels in his blood components, but mineral levels as well. Drips were administered accordingly. It brought it home to me just what a finely tuned mechanism our bodies are, how much expertise was going into getting H well, beating the leukaemia.

I was still angry about the norovirus. But my thought processes had moved on from lavender oil and lemon juice. What if the bug hadn't been picked up on the ward? I won a prize in a murder mystery weekend once – no, I wasn't planning the perfect murder! – but this was a mystery which needed solving, to avoid it happening again.

My mind settled on the parents' kitchen, frequently a mess with far too many transient, traumatised families passing through. Penny, crashing through skyscraper... It wasn't the kitchen, grotty though it could be, a hand written sign Cellotaped to a cupboard admonishing people who didn't clear up. I knew who'd written it - no, not me. It was the fridge. The fridge was filthy.

Next time I saw Daffodil Yellow I told her my theory. Her face went pale, she made her excuses and left the room. I had my answer. No one ever cleaned out the fridge. We never got on quite as well after that...

Each day felt like it was becoming more of a struggle, but each day H was improving, his bloods were responding. He had CT scans, Echo scans on his heart, anti this and anti that. Yet again I was trying to feed him without access to a fridge or a kitchen. Magda and Pops were getting on with things, but Pops' tears at night were really getting to me. She'd had enough. It was a tough call for Magda.

I didn't feel we had reached a point when I could leave him at night. Why on earth anyone within hospital management ever thought that would be possible I have no idea. Staffing levels were so tight I believed there would have been times when he would not have been cleaned up or he really could have choked on sick. I had only clocked two sets of parents who chose not to stay with their children at night.

One couple left their son, around H's age, a couple of nights, but when he went downhill, they changed their minds. He wasn't on the ward for very long.

In one of the isolation rooms there was a very young baby boy. He cried a lot, staff often had to cuddle him at night, to calm him down. The crying was awful, night after night. I couldn't understand why a parent would abandon their baby like that. He was so ill. I saw them one day; they were teenagers and the baby had Down's. It was none of my business. Each parent coped however they could; it was not my place to make value judgements about anybody else's life.

I began to take more solace in shopping. It was still a novelty being able to buy clothes and with Pops togged up it meant I could buy some stuff for myself. I was discovering the city centre shops and revelled in being two dress sizes smaller. Maybe I should send the first straight jacket back, order a smaller one?

Among the weekend carers for Pops was my other primary school buddy and official oldest friend, Katie P, and her other half Sal. They brought a breath of air to our beleaguered set up. I still marvelled that so many people were still in the loop with us, despite their own busy lives, full on jobs, families.

H's plight had touched many lives, he'd even made it onto a prayer chain in Haiti through an incredible network of Churches, starting in our home town. Many of the churches which had prayed for H were now praying for the three million people devastated by the earthquake last month. Everywhere there are circles within circles.

My dad was now off the ventilator, but I felt certain mum would never have another real conversation with him, even if he made it home. Other grandma had, true to form, pitched up in Bristol, unannounced. I think she was lonely with her husband in hospital.

I had to stay focused on the idea that each day we lived through was going to bring us one day nearer home.

'*One day at a time. Now repeat after me...*' Said Inner Goddess. '*One day at a time...*'

CHAPTER
FIFTY-TWO

I STILL CAN'T REMEMBER QUITE HOW IT HAPPENED. WELL, I CAN. WHAT I suppose I mean is 'why' it happened. Though sometimes there simply is no 'why'.

One moment I was standing in the queue in at our favourite food hall, buying a microwave meal for one, lemonade for H, a treat for Pops. I'd picked the slow queue, the one where a price is queried or the package was bust. Don't people work this out BEFORE they get in the queue?

I noticed another till open up and darted towards it; two people beat me to it. We were standing alongside the drinks section. Before I even realised the spirits were on the bottom shelf I'd sidled over, grabbed a bottle of vodka and put it in my basket. There was no thought process. There was no dithering. I just did it.

I paid, in a bit of daze, and walked back to the hospital, dashed up the stairs (must be quite fit by now) all the while wondering what on earth I was going to do with a bottle of vodka. It was a dry ward.

By the quiet of the evening, just H and I, the ward winding down for the night, I realised I'd have to do something with the bottle; the illegal, forbidden contraband. Knowing it was not allowed made it even more appealing. Why couldn't I have bought chocolate? Knowing it was there made me really want it. I must have subconsciously wanted it else I would never have bought it.

I rang Pops to say goodnight and it left me feeling bereft, helpless and angry at the situation we had been forced into. I spotted the cartons of orange juice on the window sill by H's bed. It was too much. I offered H one. He shook his head. I opened a carton and poured the juice into my clean mug, which I had taken to keeping on the window sill. I undid the screw top of the 'illegal' vodka bottle, shielding it with one of the breeding cloth bags. I double checked no one could see and poured it into the mug, along with the orange juice. By the time I was sat down on the non-reclining recliner the bottle was safely stashed in the bag under my chair.

The mug sat on the window sill for a while. I couldn't quite believe I'd done it. How much trouble would I be in if the staff found out? Would they be able to smell it?

My irrational mind figured, now it was poured, I may as well drink it, so I did. I felt it snake down my throat, the alcoholic burn offset by the overly sweet orange juice, which made its strength bearable. I took another slug. Then another. Before I knew it, the mug was empty.

I felt the warm glow. It felt so good I repeated the entire process, all the while wondering what would happen if I got caught. By the time I'd finished the second mug I knew it was time to get my bed down, while I still could. I must have giggled a bit, H asked what I was up to.

We read for a bit, him to me. A nurse came and took H's vitals. She asked me what was up – oh my goodness, it must be written all over my face! H and I both giggled, we pointed to the book. Had H twigged? Nurse laughed. It was Dr Seuss, fried green onions or something, not Cat in the Hat. 'They're great those books' she said, and with a laugh she was gone.

H was soon asleep and I was (possibly) in a quandary. But by then I was so pissed all reason had gone. For a start I would never normally drink vodka with over-sweetened orange juice, essence of cardboard a bonus. Regardless, I poured another large one and drank it.

It was the best night's sleep I'd had in ages. I even managed to make it to the communal loo at the top of the ward, without falling over. Quite a feat actually, being legless. I did manage to get tangled up in my knickers though. I just took them off and shoved them under my pillow. At least I think I did, that would have been a shock for the cleaner, it wasn't THAT kind of institution

The following morning ... oh yes, the following morning... I felt as bad as I deserved to feel. It wasn't just the raging thirst and the shakes. It was the guilt. What if something had happened during the night – to H or Pops? Would I have behaved like their mother, or a drunk?

I was so determined it should not happen again I decided, in my even more irrational, hungover, state that the only way to ensure it did not happen again was to get rid of the rest of bottle. So I did. Down my neck.

By the time Pops had arrived back from school that morning the whole bottle was gone and I was doing an impression of someone with a very bad headache which, by then, really wasn't much of an impression. Luckily, I had post swine flu Paracetamol in my bag.

When you live in the close confines of a hospital ward people notice things all the time. They just don't always notice the right things. I was tired and emotional, as were so many of the other parents. I just happened to be tired and emotional for different reasons that day.

In the afternoon Pops opted for a Burger King and I reverted to bog standard tired and emotional mum. The moment I took the empty vodka bottle out of the cloth bag dangling from my shoulder and sheepishly shoved it into a public bin – having successfully smuggled it out of the hospital - I felt like the biggest failure ever. I hope no one saw me though the clunk of the empty bottle as it hit the bottom of the metal bin seemed ever so loud. I hadn't even bothered to recycle.

I'd failed to cope. Failed to resist an urge. Failed to say no. I'd failed at being a responsible mum. I determined that was to be the end of it. Goddess-in-hiding must be enticed back again.

Once again, I can't help feeling I am in line for the 'Best Bad Mother of The Year' Award.

'And here she is,' Graham Norton trills across the airwaves (or Davina or Alan Carr or Jonathan Ross, Claudia, Fern, well, choose your award ceremony host.) 'The Best Bad Mother of the Year - for the tenth year running, she's not giving up her crown easily ...'

No sequinned dress or stilettos for me. Just the white jacket, sequins pending.

And an empty bottle.

CHAPTER
FIFTY-THREE

We were on the move again. H's norovirus meant we couldn't continue staying in CLIC House. We had little notice. I didn't get an opportunity to pack and with no car I began to panic about what on earth I was going to do.

Magda had a week's holiday because it was half term and Hayley from Devon suggested she look after Pops for a few days; they had family in Bristol who were due a visit.

Instead of calling people and asking for help I muddled through, not able to think through a plan. I packed and carried what I could. No one gave me a deadline so I assumed I had a couple of days. H was improving but the intensity of his treatment didn't abate.

By the time I picked up a message telling me the rest of our stuff at CLIC House had been bundled up into black plastic bags, left on the top floor landing, could I come and collect them *yesterday*. I was on my knees.

I was also on my high horse.

Poor Jamie got the full brunt of my raging.

'It's inhuman, just piling it all up and abandoning our stuff. What did they think I was going to do? Don't they know I haven't got a car? Why didn't someone tell me, instead of just leaving a message which I never got?'

I wasn't even in an enclosed space but was striding along a hospital corridor. No need to imagine the funny looks.

A combination of crap communication, me not asking anyone for help and being so close to losing the plot, had ensured the cock up.

Ever the professional Jamie sat me down, calmed me down and listened. I really don't know how he was so patient with me. I guess he'd probably seen it all before. I hoped he'd seen it all before. Maybe I was simply the mother from hell.

By chance their dad rang, said he could visit later. Had Inner Goddess communed with the tricky Gods of my imaginings?

'Go on you lot, give her a break!' And they had.

Without a single complaint, their dad and Pops carried every black bin bag, box and filled cloth bag down two flights of stairs and up the driveway, loaded up his large company car and drove everything to Rhys' House, the 'home from home' next door to ... Charly's House.

He picked me up outside the hospital when they were done and whisked me up to CLIC House so I could make sure the room was clear, empty our supplies from the kitchen cupboards and fridge – clean it – and start unpacking.

I bought yet another full set of cleaning stuff and set about settling us into our new abode, which was an exact replica of Charly's House, except reversed. Even the Next furniture was identical. It messed with your head, though the boiler worked and there was no gushing tap in the kitchen.

By the end of the day, I was shattered. I knew Magda wasn't happy because there was no internet connection. It was the way she kept her other life going, the life she would go back to when H was finally discharged. But we had no choice.

I hoped it meant I would have a few days with H and Pops

after he finished this third round of chemo, before he started the fourth and final one. A 'second Christmas', without snow and presents. Us three, full fridge, telly and long walks. It was a great city for walking, the architecture and parks in our location were glorious. And we had discovered the cosmopolitan Gloucester Road, packed full of charity shops, ethnic food stores and New Age frippery.

And that is exactly what happened. H was declared in remission for a third time and we were given time out for good behaviour.

We slept, ate, shopped and watched films. One day the sun shone so brightly, it was warm enough to be outside in February. H and Pops made a tent in the courtyard garden, using the washing line and a pile of blankets and scarves.

Was winter relinquishing its hold? H was as hairless as all the other cutesy kids on cancer posters. Pops followed me everywhere.

I was thrilled to hear them bickering.

CHAPTER FIFTY-FOUR

H AND I ARRIVED ON WARD 34 WITH REGULATION REFUGEE BAGS AND bedding, ready to be shown to a bed, braced for the fourth and final round of chemotherapy.

We were shown to bed 10, the one in a corner all by itself, sandwiched between the outer wall and the public bathroom. It was early March. The sun was shining and even Inner Goddess was optimistic. Until we got told to close the big glass doors.

'You're not allowed to open the doors,' said a uniformed someone.

Inner one grumped off, mumbling something about *'bloody bureaucracy, it was only a bit of fresh air...*

We unpacked and made up the beds. I was trying to keep stuff levels to a minimum. It mounts up by a hospital bed. Each bed was allocated a narrow five shelved cupboard but with drugs and living essentials, like clean knickers and sewing bags, it's not hard to accumulate more than you can carry. And visitors bring 'stuff' with them, to help make things better ...

I have always been a 'nester'; it's the Piscean, home-comfort loving side of my personality. Some people might call it hoarding.

Here in hospital, I'd developed an alter ego – the *obsessive compulsive collector.* Everything had to have a place, even when there was nowhere to put anything. I'd become a bag lady in Bristol. Everywhere I went I had at least one cloth bag on my left shoulder, constantly moving bits of stuff from A to B, and back again. Always carrying clean washing, trying to second guess the next 24 hours.

H and I prepared ourselves for the waiting to start all over again. The ward felt calm. There weren't too many people about.

Magda and Pops came for lunch, eaten by the bedside. Magda and I had got the catering pretty much sussed. We'd talk about what we'd have, I'd usually buy supplies and we juggled cooking, depending on who was where at what time of the day. Magda was both capable and practical.

We both relished our morning coffee in The Wild Wood. During those times Magda talked more of her own life. The relationship with her ex had been re-kindled and he came to visit, cooked us all cauliflower cheese. They were both talking about leaving the caring profession behind, fulfilling an ambition, opening a classy beach café, inspired by The Wild Wood – and they'd found one back in Devon!

You know the form by now. Five days of chemo, intimate knowledge of the sluice room, close monitoring, tears before bedtime, sewing for sanity.

Within days H looked very ill. His temperature spiked and we were moved back into Room 4. He had a non-specific infection. Round four sapped him and he started getting uncharacteristically grumpy with doctors and nurses. Out of frustration he bit me, hard on my arm, during a doctor's visit. He glared at me and all I could see was his weariness. H had shown nothing but bravery. He was done in, after almost five months of hideous treatments.

Pops also, by that stage, had had enough. One morning I had to give both her and Magda a talking to. There was an atmosphere between them which had become unsettling. Somehow, I found a way of talking to a seven-year-old as if she was a thirty-something and a thirty-something as if she was not a seven-year-old.

'I hope I still know you away from here,' said Magda. I took it as an endorsement, that I had managed to find the right words. Words, by then, didn't matter to Pops.

One day I broke down in front of Lovely Zoe, confessed I didn't know how much longer I could cope with Pops sobbing down the phone every night. She was very kind, but listening didn't change anything.

Talking to Pops on the phone the following evening – by then she had her own, child-friendly mobile and rang me frequently, even when Magda told her not to – I snapped.

H was off chemo. He'd finished his anti-fungal for the day and he was dressed. I rang a taxi and, as we were walking out of the ward Lovely Zoe saw us.

'Where are you going?' she asked, sharply.

'To spend the night with my daughter,' I said, equally sharply.

'You can't take H with you,' she said.

'Yes, I can', I said. And I did.

I felt we'd just become fugitives, on the run from the law. I had no idea I had, in reality, sparked a security alert.

Senior management was alerted as we drove away from the hospital back to Rhys' House, to be greeted by a thrilled Pops and a confused Magda.

Had the hospital team not been able to raise Jamie, who said, in his judgement, I would not do anything to endanger H, the police would have been called. If the police had arrived to escort me and H back to hospital, I would have grabbed both my children and run away through the back door. That is not an exaggeration. The pressure had got to me and I was irrational, fight and flight mode combined. I would have run.

Magda was concerned, but I was adamant I was staying. When the children were asleep Magda, wonderful Magda, calmed me down and we put together a plan. She had slept at the hospital a couple of nights. When H was well, she would take on more of his care and I would spend more nights with Pops.

H and I returned to hospital the following morning, in time for his morning bloods. One look from Jamie told me how much trouble I was in.

'We do know the pressure you're under,' he said, 'but you can't do that again. You know that, don't you?'

My defiance evaporated. I apologised. He softened.

'How do you keep going Sharon? We can all see how hard this is for you' he said.

'Same way everyone else does,' I said. 'Thanks Jamie. I promise I won't do it again. We all just want to go home.'

I'd had a major bollocking, without Jamie verbalising the seriousness of what I'd done. Jamie should have been nominated for a Knighthood, dealing with a mum like me.

Inner Goddess remained defiant, determined to escape for real at the earliest possible opportunity.

Inner Goddess's weaker sister bought another bottle of vodka. The shame of it was far worse than the first. But it took the edge off, clouded reality. I dodged reality when I could. It got me through the next couple of weeks. Did anyone know? Magda must have. I didn't care by then.

I missed two funerals during round four of H's chemotherapy.

Other granddad died, in hospital, of a brain tumour. I tried very hard to sort a hire car and dash down to Plymouth, but H and Pops needed me more. I know he would have understood.

My friend Val, who prepared me more for cancer in the week we three had spent with her in France than anything else could ever have done. She died of breast cancer. Even if I'd had my passport in Bristol, I could not have left H and Pops. I know she would also have understood.

Two funerals snapped me out of the self-pity.

Plans to leave hospital emerged.

It was terrifying. It felt more terrifying than staying.

CHAPTER
FIFTY-FIVE

H was finally discharged from Bristol Children's Hospital on April 1st 2010.

The joke was not lost on us.

Inner Goddess thought it was hilarious.

Someone in the top floor day clinic said 'they've made an appointment for you...' The appointment was for the day before we were due to drive back to Devon, the day a friend was driving my car up. The someone gave me a scrap of paper, with the name *Bramble Ward* written on it, and a phone number with a code I didn't know. I had no idea which hospital Bramble Ward was actually in. I rang the number. No one answered.

CHAPTER FIFTY-SIX

ABSEIL

We were sitting on Budleigh Salterton beach. Not a beach of nostalgic holiday snaps depicting little ones building sandcastles, discovering the feel of sea water, ice creams dripping. It is a beach of large pebbles, smooth to the hand but rough on the feet.

H and Pops were pottering near the water's edge. We have never swum there; deep shelves and foot rough slopes don't make it very friendly. Yet it is a glorious beach, the history of buildings which once housed ancient mariners and wealthy sea faring families oozes gently into the atmosphere.

It was Katie P who first took me there, years before children and grown-up stuff. We wandered in an October rain mist, licked ice cream while we sat in her car and revelled in our freedom.

Many years on and it is the day before school returns after the summer holidays. Pops will go back. H will, but not every day. He is still being home tutored.

I watched my children; seemingly happy, unfettered, showing no signs of any particular illness. Every moment felt precious. Because it was.

The posters in my handbag were bugging me.

The CLIC Sargent Abseil.

Cantonteign Falls

Saturday September 25 2010

Several of our home town shops had put posters in their windows. I felt I'd done *'my bit'* by asking them. Yet I couldn't get the thought out of my head; I should do the abseil. If H could endure almost six months of hell to come home in remission, surely, I could dangle on the end of a bit of rope for a few minutes. I loved water. I'm a natural fish. Surely, I could cope with the highest waterfall in England. A mere 220 feet. Or was it the thought of having to squeeze into a wet suit which put me off?

Oh for goodness sake, laughed the woman inside. *Are you really that scared of a bit of neoprene squeezing your arse into something tight?*

Driving home from the beach, I mulled. I'm sure people would sponsor me to do it. It would take some effort. Could I persuade a friend to do it with me? Light bulb moment – Sarah! She was fit, active and courageous. I could ask her. But could I do it? Was I brave enough?

What did I have to lose by asking? So I did. I figured if she said 'no' then I was off the hook. It was a bit of a shocker when she said 'OK!'.

I suppose we talked each other into it. We filled out the forms, calculated we could raise enough to meet requirements (all charity dare devil events require a minimum sponsorship to cover costs). There was no way out.

As the date got closer, I think we both realised what a huge undertaking we were now involved with. Not just the abseil itself, but raising sponsorship. Neither of us had partner back up. We both worked. As the day drew nearer it was the thought of the deed itself which began to freak me out. Sarah seemed calm. I kept telling myself she was physically fit and would look great in a wet suit, with her slinky, model-girl looks.

Me, well, 'I-knew-I-was-going-to-look-rubbish-in-a-wet-suit-and-I-haven't-been-in-the-gym-enough-lately'. That's my look. I never need to ask, 'does my bum look big in this?'

H and Pops were excited, but had picked up on my nerves. I drove us there and parked up, meeting a clutch of wonderful friends, including Sarah's mum, dad and daughter, Pops' bestie. We got to the entrance and I was asked to pay before the children were allowed to go in.

CLIC Sargent had already alluded to this scenario and both Sarah and I had asked the area fundraiser if it was true. We were told we were on our own.

The woman on the gate eventually let H in for free, when I pointed out I was fundraising for children like him who had been treated for cancer. I had to pay for Pops. I couldn't dwell on the irony of it all, the 'I'm raising money for people like us' - yet we had to pay to be there.

I had to move on. I was about to tackle the highest waterfall in England. In a wet suit. I really shouldn't be allowed out on my own some days. This was one of them. Please, helicopter in a straight jacket, pretty please.

We sat in the café. Julia and fiancé Russ arrived; friends made on Ward 34. It was brilliant to see them. Russ had raised thousands to do the abseil, so he'd won a camera to be fitted on his helmet, recording the experience. I felt lucky to get a helmet which almost fitted. I have a small head, which of course makes my body look so much bigger, particularly in a wet suit, even though it was black.

Was it just me or did the abseil crew look very young in a devil-may-care kind of way? Other abseilers were lining up, we all had time slots. There had obviously been group 'dares' going on, people had come from miles around to take part, some were wearing pink tutus. It was all very *gung ho.* All I wanted to do was run.

The 'lad' fitting my harness expressed surprise it was my first ever abseil.

'I thought they liked people to have had some experience before tackling this one,' he said.

'I did fill in the questionnaire, saying it was my first' I said, not quite managing a smile.

Even Sarah admitted she was 'a bit nervous'.

'It's fine,' I said to H and Pops. 'Let's do it!'

I was still hanging on to the idea if H could do what he'd done, endured almost six months without complaining, I could do this one small thing.

We started walking up the hill to get to the top of the waterfall. Marbles. All gone. Mouth dry. Toilet too far away and, quite frankly, not an option in the wet suit. It may as well have been Everest.

I felt sick. Sick at the thought of doing it. Sick at the thought of not doing it, facing the humiliation of always being known in town as the 'woman who chickened out'.

Please certify me now. Please wake me up, this must be a nightmare. I couldn't see any of the beauty around me. The stunning landscape, trees still green, about to embrace autumn, the waterfall itself, which you could hear before it came into view. Two hundred and twenty foot of water gushing down a rocky cliff face makes quite a noise. Or was that just the rushing inside my head?

This is for H.

This is for H.

This is for H.

You can do it.

You can do it.

You can do it.

Hadn't I had enough fear? Why was I so stupid? I had nothing to prove? Just turn around and walk away, bleated a voice in my head.

'How dare you!' said Inner Goddess. *'This is a small thing in the universe and you will keep your promise. Up you go.'*

Another meaningless pep talk, from bloke at the top. Sarah was over the metal railings and away. She was doing it. She was amazing. She was down. So was the short mousey woman before me. She was doing it for someone, I can't remember who.

I wasn't sure how I was going to get over the railings as by then I had no sensation in either of my arms.

'The first step is the hardest,' said bloke manning the railings.

'Come on, you can do it,' he said, the ring distinctly hollow.

My children were watching from the bottom, as were our friends. Sarah was down. Sarah was safe. I had to. No way out.

'This will be over soon,' said voice in head.

'It will never be over if you don't do it', said Inner Goddess. *'Come on love,'* she said, sounding softer. *'You really can do this'.*

I climbed over the railings.

Clipped to my harness was a bit of coloured, high tech rope. Let's hope the outdoorsy blokes knew their knots. Would it hold me? Was there a load limit on the rope? I hadn't thought to ask, until it was too late.

The tag line for the event was *'A Lifeline for Children with Cancer'.* That rope has suddenly become the only thing anchoring me to this world.

'It's a bit tricky this bit. That's it. Feet nice and wide,' said Outdoors Bloke.

'That's great. Well done. Now remember how to let out the rope, that's it. Feet wide,' he said.

I had blank mind syndrome. My feet were spread on a piece of rubber mat. Don't look down. Look at the rocks. One step at a time. My foot couldn't grip anything, it was so slippery. I tried to remember the 'training'. By that I mean the fifteen-minute pep talk when you get to fiddle with your harness and let out the rope attached to a thingy on your bum. While standing on the ground.

The water was coming at me and I there was only one way to go.

Physically I could never have climbed back over the railings.

Stay calm.

Think of H and Pops.

Running away not allowed.

I thought back to the day of diagnoses, that Sunday morning when H had been crying out in pain, stuck on the stairs.

This fear could not possibly be worse than that.

Do it.

I moved my feet wider, leaned away from the rope, felt the tension, let the rope out, bit by bit, began walking backwards.

Breathe. OK, don't, you'll drown. Water in my face.

Stay calm.

Spring off the rocks with your feet, let the rope out, slowly.

Do it.

I was terrified.

Fight the fear. Breathe.

I made it to the halfway point, to be greeted by another Outdoorsy Bloke standing in a pool of water created by a natural rock formation. He was placed to give encouragement to weary abseilers. Talk them down to the bottom of the waterfall.

'Get your breath back' he said. I was hyperventilating. The water was icy cold.

'This is the hardest one we do. It's pretty challenging,' he said. Was that meant to be reassuring?

'Your first one?' I managed to nod.

'Oh,' he said.

I was beyond speech. Got my breath back, set off again.

Had to get this over with. Didn't think the rescue helicopter, which was not in attendance, would have been able to land on such a small ledge on the face of a waterfall.

It felt as if it was inch by inch, but it must have been foot by foot.

As I got a bit further down, I could hear something. Bit further. It got louder. *Come on girl, they're all here for you,* said Inner Goddess. I span round, couldn't get a grip on the rocks which were covered in green slippery stuff. My head seemed to be spinning. It WAS spinning. I couldn't get a grip, couldn't right myself, couldn't move down. I had no control. OMG, was I upside down? I crashed into the rocks, my left thigh throbbed, despite the freezing cold water it really hurt.

Think H. How much he had endured. You'll get a piffling bruise. So what!

If I didn't get a better position, I was going to carry on swallowing water and I was beginning to choke, I couldn't breathe. If I die here there is no one who can look after H and Pops. That thought was enough. I found the strength, my arms pulled me up. Was that angel feathers brushing my numb cheek? Or was I hallucinating?

Get a grip, shouted Inner Goddess.

I'm bloody trying, I shouted back.

The noise was louder. It was shouting. No, it was cheering.

Few more inches... What do you mean it's all metric now? I was stressed, I was thinking in imperial, give me a break!

The cheering was getting louder. I realised the cheering was for me. I could hear my name; they were chanting my name. Few more feet.

Legs hit stone. It was a slimy ledge. Surely I must be nearly down. Instinctively I looked round. I could see rocks spreading out below me. I was nearly there! The cheering was louder than the crashing water. I swivelled. I could see H and Pops. Just a few more feet. This was easy.

I shoved my feet off from the rocks and let go too much rope, juddered to the ground. Knees – who needs 'em? I was on slippery solid ground.

I didn't walk over to the cheering group, I wobbled. I was engulfed and my children had their arms around me first.

'Mummy! Mummy! You've done it,' said H. 'You were brilliant!'

'Was it scary?' said Pops. 'You're all wet!'

'Even my knickers are soaked,' I said, much to their disapproval.

'Did you realise you were hanging upside down at one point,' said Sarah. 'That was really scary to watch. God I'm glad that's over. H was cheering louder than anyone else,' she said. 'He was jumping up and down, like he was willing you down.'

I passed Inner Goddess a soggy tissue. We all walked down the hill. On the way up I'd missed the magic in the mossy rocks and ancient trees.

On the way down I drank it in, a child's hand in each of mine.

When I wrote all this, I had no way of knowing ten years and one day after discharge, life would get much tougher. I had sequins and I could still thread a needle ...

Acknowledgments

I wrote this book for three very specific reasons: to raise awareness of childhood cancer, to say thank you to everyone who helped and guided us through the trauma and got H well – especially all the remarkable nurses and doctors on Ward 34, as well as Lin, Jamie and Magda - and to ensure H and Pops know I continue to be proud of the authentic people they are becoming.

So many people, so many people in our home towns, have their place in Sewing Sequins on My Straight Jacket. I hope every one of you appreciates all you have done for us. A heartfelt THANK YOU for all your kindness and support.

To reach the point of publication takes more than writing a book, which as any writer knows is quite some process, taking a not inconsiderable dash of madness and bloody- minded determination.

I am indebted to my first writing buddy, Kate and her husband Michael, my current writing buddy Margaret and her husband Chris (AKA Chef), to Sandra (and Alan!), The Evening Stars, Lizzie, Katie P and Sal, Becky and Jayne. Without the final push from crime writer Val Penny, Nikki and Sumira of Spell-Bound - and Teen Cancer nurse Lorraine - Sewing Sequins on My Straight Jacket would never have left the drawer I dumped it in ...

I hope this book helps others, and gets some conversations started.

And if pushed for advice – don't buy the cheap tissues, unless you want to get covered in snot.

Printed in Great Britain
by Amazon

48649279R00179